Mother and Daughter

Mother and Daughter

(No More Soup)

Louise Joy

iUniverse, Inc.
New York   Bloomington

Mother and Daughter
(No More Soup)

iUniverse books may be ordered through booksellers or by contacting:

iUniverse
1663 Liberty Drive
Bloomington, IN 47403
www.iuniverse.com
1-800-Authors (1-800-288-4677)

Because of the dynamic nature of the Internet, any Web addresses or links contained in this book may have changed since publication and may no longer be valid. The views expressed in this work are solely those of the author and do not necessarily reflect the views of the publisher, and the publisher hereby disclaims any responsibility for them.

ISBN: 978-1-4401-2625-3 (sc)
ISBN: 978-1-4401-2626-0 (ebook)

Printed in the United States of America

iUniverse rev. date: 2/25/2009

This book is dedicated to my father and husband, who both showed courage and strength in facing their destiny and who both lost their battle with cancer, at home, with dignity, surrounded by family.

They were loved, are loved and will never be forgotten.

Table of Contents

INTRODUCTION

Yes, I can attest that truth is stranger than fiction. My life is living proof that no one can predict their future. You can plan, dream and wish upon a star but if fate has other plans for you there is no rhyme or reason for the sequence of events that happen in your life. After reading this book, you will understand why I truly feel that when it's your time to leave this earthly world, you will have no control over the outcome, no matter what you do, what resources are available or how hard you pray. It doesn't matter. When your time is up, there are no other choices.

If you get nothing else from the following pages, at the very least, I hope you gain the knowledge that you must enjoy every day and not let one minute pass you by. Say what you mean, mean what you say and be careful what you wish for. Tell your families you love them and cherish all the fun and wonderful moments you share together, for you will never know and can never predict when it could be your last minute together. Life can change in a day, in an hour, or in a minute.

Never live in the past or dwell on what you can't change but rather live in the moment and grasp and make every minute count in your life. Make sure you bond with your immediate and extended families, including parents, brothers, sisters, grandparents, cousins, aunts and uncles. Always look for the good in people because when the earth falls from beneath your feet, family ties and bonds as well as good friends are what holds it together and helps to get you through.

CHAPTER ONE

GROWING UP

I grew up an only child in Staten Island, New York with two loving parents. My father worked in the construction field and when I started school my mother went back to work as a teller in one of the local banks. My childhood was fairly normal. My maternal grandfather lived on the same block, two houses down. He was a widower and had lost his wife when my mother was only twenty-one years old and before she was married. My mother had a brother twelve years older and a sister ten years older. They were both already married when my grandmother died. I regret not knowing my maternal grandmother. I'm sure it would have been nice to have her around when I was growing up. My grandfather was very self-sufficient and over the years had learned to cook for himself and a very good cook he was. He had a huge back yard and an amazing garden. As a child, I remember walking down rows of planted tomatoes, corn and strawberries as well as many other vegetables. He had a green thumb for sure.

I attended a Catholic grammar school which very conveniently was located across the street from where I lived. In those days you were allowed to go home for lunch if you lived nearby so some days I would walk across the street and have lunch at my grandfather's house when my mother was at work.

When I was eleven years old, we moved into a brand new two-family house which my parents had custom built. They had bought a piece of property and I remember the architect coming to the house and drawing up the plans for our new home. Working in the construction field afforded my father the knowledge to oversee and hire contractors he knew and also be able to do a lot of the work himself. When the house was finished, my parents and I moved in upstairs and my maternal grandfather moved in downstairs. Little did I know the future that I or the rest of us would have in our new home. After the move, I also transferred to a junior high school in my area. I kept my old friends and also made friends in my new neighborhood and my new school.

When I was twelve years old, my paternal grandmother died after an operation she had for cancer. She never drank or smoked but suffered from cancer of the voice box. The surgery was successful but a blood clot to her lung killed her. It was the first wake and funeral I had ever attended. It was scary and I remember telling my mother that I didn't want to go up to the coffin but she said I had to. So, I made my way up, kissed my grandmother on the cheek and I remember her skin feeling very hard and cold. I also remember the drive in the limo the morning of her funeral. As we were driving to the cemetery, my grandfather was crying. Certain moments in your life are unforgetable.

Marriage and Children

As I grew into my teens, I had all of the usual dreams and aspirations of a normal teenager. The typical dream of meeting my "Prince Charming" galloping up on his white horse and sweeping me away to live happily ever after was always ever present. Also in my dream was the desire to have children. Five to be exact was the number of children I always wished to have. Since I was an only child, I longed to have a big family.

After high school, I went to business school and then went to work in Manhattan in the secretarial field. That was in the seventies which was also the disco era. Dancing in the discos every weekend was the _"in thing."_ It was a good and fun time in my life which included dating, going out with friends and searching for _"Mr. Right!"_ Well, the years went by and I was now in my twenties. When I was twenty-five, I met my "Prince Charming." He wasn't riding on a white horse but rather dressed in blue. He was a New York City police officer who also worked as a bouncer in a bar in Manhattan on his nights off. He had his own apartment in New York City and a mutual friend had introduced us.

We just seemed to hit it off and after two weeks of dating, he popped the question. Of course everyone's reaction was the same. "It's too soon. You don't even know each other. Give it some time." But, I was twenty-five and he was twenty-seven and we just knew it was right. So, we got engaged, made our plans and ten months later in September of 1980, we were married. We had a beautiful honeymoon in Bermuda. Life was good.

Of course, when you come home from the honeymoon, reality sets in. It's back to a work schedule as well as all the responsibilities of married life. In addition to your job, you are responsible for cooking, cleaning, food shopping, doing the laundry and all the other fun chores that go along with marriage. My husband had given up his apartment in the city to move to Staten Island. We lived in a one-bedroom apartment and at least once a week we would go to my parent's house for dinner or visit on the weekend. Sometimes I would bring the laundry at the same time since, as apartment dwellers, we didn't have the convenience of a washer and dryer.

My husband and I were also from different ethnic backgrounds. He was Jewish and I am an Italian Catholic. However, it didn't matter to us. We were compatible and never let religion affect our lives. After two years of marriage our son was born. He had ruby red lips and a full head of black hair. After he was born, I stopped working to be a full time mom. Two years and four months later we were also blessed with a daughter. She was fair skinned and bald but beautiful just the same. She had blue eyes just like my father's. We had the perfect family, a boy, a girl and eventually a dog, a golden retriever named Candi. We were in agreement to raise the children Catholic and religion was never an issue in our home. We celebrated all the holidays and both traditions. My husband loved the holidays and having family around.

Family Life

My father had retired from construction in the late 1970's and was now working as a grinder, a trade he had learned from his father when he was a young boy. He had bought a truck which he equipped and customized himself and went neighborhood to neighborhood both in Staten Island and Brooklyn, ringing the bell, sharpening scissors, knives and many other tools. Among his regular customers were some of the gardeners and landscapers in our borough. My father was a perfectionist in his trade and was also very fair in his prices. He was well respected for his excellent work and also for the good and fair person that he was.

My father would come home with stories of the day. One time, he sharpened knives for a gay man who had invited my father in for some pie he had just baked. My father politely declined. Then there was also the time he had sharpened several scissors and knives for tenants in an apartment building in Brooklyn. As he was going up the stairwell to deliver the sharpened tools, he was stopped and surrounded by police with their guns drawn. Someone in the building had called the police having reported a man carrying knives in the building! When the police realized he was just the grinder doing his job, they laughed and put their guns away. Also, when small children would hear the bell they would run up to the truck thinking he was the ice cream man.

My son was three and my daughter eight months old when my husband and I lost our remaining three grandparents. It happened during the summer of 1985. My maternal grandfather died in June, my husband's paternal grandmother died in July and my paternal grandfather died in August. But the one that impacted me the most was when my maternal grandfather died. He was the one who had lived downstairs in my house and who I was the closest to. He was ninety-six years old and had lived a good and pretty healthy life. He had suffered a stroke and only lasted a few days in the hospital. But, up until the day of his stroke, he was still cooking for himself, able to walk to the store everyday and even took the bus to get his haircuts. I know that no one lives forever and he was after all ninety-six, but I really missed him. He was very good to me and he loved my children very much. He used to play with them and hold them and just loved when I brought them over to visit. His passion had always been his garden. That was his hobby and he used to work in the garden for hours. I would miss that too. As I stated earlier, he was also a great cook; having taught himself after his wife had died. He made the best sauce and pasta fagioli. He used to also drink half a glass of wine mixed with half of cream soda with his lunch every day. Mixing wine with soda is a custom of some Italians and when he was low on wine he would ask my husband to buy him another gallon to which my husband was always happy to oblige.

After things settled down, my mother and father asked me and my husband if we wanted to move in and live upstairs. Since there were three bedrooms upstairs and my mother and father didn't need all that room for just the two of them, they said they would renovate my grandfather's apartment and move downstairs. Raising a family on a police officer's salary did not afford us a lot of luxuries and I wasn't working at the time because my children were still babies. Trying to save for a house was almost impossible and this was a wonderful opportunity. I was, after all, an only child, so what could be better.

By the time the renovation downstairs was completed and we were able to move into my parent's house, my daughter had just turned one and my son was three years old. We moved in a few weeks before Christmas and I had everything unpacked and the Christmas tree up and decorated before the holiday arrived. Looking back, I don't know how I did it.

After a couple of years, I was offered a job opportunity from friends who owned their own business, with the flexibility to work in their office a few hours at a time whatever days I was available, doing secretarial work. I spoke it over with my husband, since my daughter was only three years old and not in school yet. However, my son was now in kindergarten and we decided that a few hours a day, a few days a week would be okay. My husband was now working as a Community Affairs Officer on Staten Island as he had transferred to Staten Island from the Manhattan precinct he was working in right after our son was born. His hours rotated and a few days a week he worked afternoon to evening hours depending on what community meetings he needed to attend. So, on those days, I went to work a few hours in the morning, which meant he would be able to be at home with our daughter. At least if any problems arose that my husband needed help with, my mother was right downstairs and she had offered to help out as well. It was an ideal situation and as time went on and my daughter started preschool, my days and hours increased so that I worked a few days a week the hours both my children were in school. I drove them to school in the morning, went to work, then picked them up after school. I also had the flexibility to change a work day if there was a school function I needed to attend or if one of the children were sick and I needed to take them to the doctor or be at home with them. I didn't miss out on a thing when they were in grammar school. My husband even arranged school trips for their classes to the local precinct where he worked.

Vacations and Holidays

Like most families, we took vacations every summer with our kids. We usually went to the Poconos in Pennsylvania and over the years vacationed at a few different resorts. Finally, one year, we got the opportunity to take a trip to Disney in Florida and had a great time. We also took a cruise to the Caribbean Islands when my daughter was fifteen. My son, then seventeen, didn't want to go. He was getting to the age where vacationing with your parents was not cool, so he remained at home with his grandparents.

My husband was also obsessed with videotaping every occasion and vacation. As the children were growing up, he would videotape the kids, set up funny scenarios and prompted them in what to say. It was amazing how his mind worked. Even our children's birthday parties were precluded with my husband interviewing them and setting the tone for the day.

My husband had also become close with my extended family of aunts, uncles and cousins. The holidays were always special and he enjoyed them tremendously. Thanksgiving was always at our house. My daughter has a karaoke machine so during the course of the day, usually before dessert, we would all take turns singing karaoke. I have my husband on tape singing along with Frank Sinatra, whom he idolized, and everyone else chiming in and having a great time. I have many videos and memories of very special times of Thanksgiving holidays at our house. My father has two sisters and Christmas Eve was always spent at one sister's house and Christmas Day was either at his other sister's house or at the home of one of my cousins.

For my son's first Christmas, my husband went out and bought a Santa Suit. He was the only Jewish Santa in the family and he did it the best. He loved to dress up and play Santa Claus for the children in the family every Christmas Eve. It became a tradition and the whole family looked forward to it every year. Inevitably, after dinner the little ones would look out the window and the adults would all prompt them by saying, "Look, can you see the lights?" "Santa is coming!" All the time, my husband would disappear upstairs to don his Santa outfit.

Sometimes he needed a little pillow for extra padding and sometimes he didn't, depending on the year and the diet. Anyway, he would come down the stairs, ringing his Santa bell and chanting, *"Merry Christmas!"* The children would get so excited and he would sit on the couch, call out the names, give out the presents and all the kids would take pictures with him as Santa. It was truly a special event.

The Fourth of July was always a barbeque at the same aunt's house where we would spend Christmas Eve. My husband always brought a patriotic tape or CD and would have them play patriotic music. One year he even made everyone stand while they played "God Bless America." Everyone, although laughing, always obliged. He was very patriotic and proud of his country.

CHAPTER TWO

LIFE AFTER RETIREMENT

As I mentioned previously, my husband had worked as a Detective in Community Affairs having also acquired the Detective shield. He was very well known and extremely popular within the community. He could get up and talk in front of a crowd of hundreds of people without being prepared. He would just talk from the heart and it would come natural. One time, he was even interviewed on a local radio station discussing an upcoming police event known as "National Night Out."

My husband retired from the police department in 1993. Upon his retirement, he had many receptions given in his honor by various community groups. Even the Borough President's office gave him a reception and a proclamation designating November 17, 1993 to be "His Official Day." At home we had a hallway full of plaques and citations from the police department as well as various groups and organizations in recognition for all his excellent work. All through the years, I had saved all kinds of memorabilia including newspaper articles, awards, pictures and letters from thankful citizens for good deeds he had performed. I compiled everything, made an album and presented it to my husband upon his retirement. It was a nice keepsake to have for all the years of hard work. He was very much admired by his peers for being a good and kind hearted person.

All through his tenure with the police department, my husband always worked a second job doing private security to make extra money. He was a good father and husband and was a straight shooter, always conscientious of doing the right thing and providing for his family. Even in his work, he gave his all, going above and beyond the job responsibility and then some.

After retiring, my husband went to work full time in the private security sector. Our children were young at the time, ages eleven and nine, so living on his police pension alone was not an option. So, as most city retirees decide, he had taken the option to get the maximum pension benefits, with the stipulation that, in case of death, his pension would cease. This, of course meant that I would receive zilch upon my husband's death. Simply put, the pension and medical insurance would die along with my husband. That's why families usually acquire life insurance, which we did, especially since our children were still young. Most city workers face these decisions upon approaching their retirement.

Summer Home

In 1994, we had purchased a summer home in the Poconos. I called it my husband's mid life crisis because it was his idea. We bought the house at a fair price since it was in foreclosure. It was a cute house with three bedrooms and a screened in porch. It was located in a community in Dingmans Ferry where some of the owners were permanent residents and others were like us and just used their residence as a summer home. One of the drawbacks was that the nearest grocery store and shopping areas were miles away. So, on our weekend trips, besides packing up the kids and the dog, I used to shop for groceries before we left so as to bring up whatever food we needed. However, most times after we arrived at our Pocono house, we would inevitably have to go miles down the road to buy milk or some other staple while we were there.

In the beginning, my husband used to say, "I just love it up here." We furnished it nicely and had obtained some new and used furniture and also had the outside of the house painted to freshen it up. We also bought a barbeque grill as well and most of the time cooked outside. However, the house was not without its problems. During the course of the summer, the septic had backed up in our back yard and we had to hire someone to pump it out and we also had mice in the house which we had to dispose of from time to time as they had inhabited the crawl space under the house. So, until we got rid of them, every once in a while we would see one run across the room and have to catch it and remove it from the house. That was after we would put the dog in one of the bedrooms so she wouldn't catch it. Then we would have to listen to the kids yelling "Don't kill it! Don't kill it!" So we would catch the mice in one of my plastic containers and then my husband would let them loose in the empty lot across the street. It was a real adventure.

We also had a community pool in our development. However, that particular summer the pool had a fungus and no one could swim in it. The teenagers who lived there all year round burned down the club house and one weekend, our neighbor's kids broke into our screened in porch. We found out after they confessed to their father, who was at least decent enough to come over and offer to pay for our broken screen door. Our neighbor on the other side of us had a black labrador retriever and right after the door was fixed and the new screen put in, the dog came up the steps and walked right through the bottom of the door and pushed in the new screen. I used to feed the dog cookies except this time he didn't wait for me to open the door and just pushed through the screen. So, needless to say, the screen had to be fixed yet once again. Yes, this was truly a home away from home. It was becoming more of a problem than it was worth.

By the end of the summer we had just about had it. My husband had now changed his tune to "I just hate it up here!" The final straw was the day he put a steak on the barbeque only to realize that there was no more gas in the tank which finally drove him over the edge. So, the grill got kicked down the hill and the keys went to a local real estate agent and the house was put up for sale. We were lucky as it didn't take long to sell. A young couple having their first child bought it to live there permanently. So, basically, we bought and sold our house within a year. So much for our summer home which literally only lasted one summer!

Getting On With Life

That same year, I was laid off from my job because a new manager was hired and decided he only wanted full time employees. I guess it didn't matter that I had worked there for seven years, but I was able to collect unemployment so I took some time off. When my unemployment benefits ended, I took an office position working for a printing company. I worked there for a couple of years and then left to start my own business. I started a printing company on my own and created a home based business consisting of wedding and all occasion invitations and also went around to the local businesses to promote the printing of business cards and stationery. I generated some local business and for a few months, I had also rented space in a discount bridal shop but it wasn't very lucrative. It was fun for a while but not having the money to invest in opening up my own store, I decided to go back to work in the secretarial field. I was hired to work for an attorney in 1999 and began a career as a legal secretary. My position was part time, working three days a week from nine to five.

As the years went by, my husband had worked his way up in the security industry and now had a prestigious position in one of the Manhattan museums as the Assistant Security Director. It was now June, 2002, my son was nineteen and my daughter was seventeen and she had just graduated from high school. My son was working for a car dealer since, after a couple of semesters in college, he decided college life was not for him. My daughter would be starting college in September. Her desire was to be a teacher. Also, since both children were now older, we had decided to downsize our life insurance policy. After all, we were doing fairly well and the kids were old enough and able to work, so we cut our life insurance by half so as to pay a smaller premium. *Big Mistake!* As we would soon find out it was not a good decision.

My husband had also started a diet about four months earlier and was looking good and feeling great. We used to like to go to Atlantic City for weekend getaways. All was well with the world, or so we thought. I could never have imagined how my world was about to be changed forever and what would be in store for all of us over the course of the next eight months.

CHAPTER THREE

<u>MY FATHER'S ILLNESS</u>

On Monday, July 1, 2002, just two days after my daughter's high school graduation party, my mother convinced my father to go to the doctor for a checkup. He had been constantly clearing his throat and felt like maybe he had a lingering cold or an allergy and had also been more tired than usual, taking a lot of naps. My mother usually went with my father to the doctor, but this time she let him go alone. My father came home and informed us that the doctor, upon checking the glands in his neck, found a lump at the base of his neck. The doctor had asked my father, "How long have you had this lump?" My father's reply was, "I didn't know I had a lump!" It wasn't something that was visible. It was under the surface of the skin. Little did we know that, at this point, our family doctor already knew that this was very serious.

Upon the doctor's instructions, my mother made an appointment for my father to go the very next day, July 2nd, to an eye, ear, nose and throat doctor to do a laryngoscope, which is a procedure where a scope is inserted through the nose and down the throat to check more extensively. Oh thank God, it was good news. The doctor said everything else from the neck up was clear. However, after that procedure, my father lost his voice. We were told by the doctors that sometimes, after a laryngoscope, your voice can be hoarse for a while. Whether or not that was really true or whether it disrupted the mass in my father's neck we were never sure but, after that test, my father would never fully regain his voice. Sometimes it was stronger than other times but it would never be the same. Most times he could only speak in a whisper.

That July 4th we went to my aunt's house as always. My father's voice was so hoarse and I remember being uneasy because every time he ate, it would irritate his throat and he would cough. It made me nervous because I was afraid he was going to choke. The only thing that seemed to soothe his throat that day was beer, believe it or not. So, he sipped beer all day.

A day or so later, it was a typical beautiful hot July summer day. We were all sitting in the back yard just relaxing by our pool. My mother decided to call their family doctor, without my father knowing, to see if she could get some information from him and ask his opinion of the lump on my father's neck. The doctor confirmed the worst. He knew the lump in my father's neck was malignant, which meant it was definitely cancerous. A doctor doesn't usually make that statement unless he is absolutely sure. How could this be? My father was never sick and had never had any kind of medical tests in his life except for a chest X-ray. He was a strong and active man. My father was also sitting outside in a chair under the canopy in the shade. As I observed him, I could actually see his mind working and sensed by his facial expression that he was talking to himself in his mind. I'm sure he must have been very scared.

After my mother's telephone conversation with the doctor, she came back outside to tell me what the doctor had said, without letting my father hear her. We didn't want to tell him anything yet or alarm him before we had all the facts and test results. It was bad enough that we could see that all kinds of thoughts were racing through his head already. After my mother told me and my husband her conversation with the doctor, she went back inside. My husband followed her in because he knew she was upset but I stayed outside and had to pretend for my father's sake that nothing was wrong. As I was sure and my husband confirmed to me later, inside the house my mother had broken down and was crying. My son, who was also in the house at the time, now heard my mother crying and came outside to ask me what was wrong. I had to quietly explain the situation and told him to act like nothing was wrong in front of his grandfather. This was a nightmare and only the beginning of horrible events to come. The panic was now starting to set in for all of us. What a mess this was becoming.

Further Medical Testing

My father still had more medical tests to be done. Before the doctors could make a definite diagnosis, he needed to have further testing done to see if the cancer had progressed anywhere else. So, on Wednesday, July 10th, my father went for a CT scan of his upper neck and chest. Then, on Wednesday, July 17th, which was also my father's seventy-fifth birthday, he had a biopsy done of the lump in his neck by a pathologist in Brooklyn who my father had been referred to by his doctor. It was done right in the pathologist's office with a needle aspiration. When we got the results, it was confirmed that it was definitely cancer cells. My father now realized that this was serious. More testing was scheduled, but before he had more tests our family doctor had already referred us to an oncologist for an initial consultation which took place on July 24th. I went with my parents to the oncologist's office for the consultation. The oncologist basically told us that the type of cancer my father had was called Adenocarcinoma. However, the oncologist also wanted more testing done to determine if there was cancer anywhere else before he would decide what protocol and regimen of chemotherapy treatment my father would need.

My father was scheduled to have a gastroscopy on Thursday, July 25th. The oncologist also wanted my father to have a colonoscopy and a CT scan of his abdomen. So, on Thursday, July 25th, my father had a gastroscopy and colonoscopy. The colonoscopy was clear but the gastroscopy revealed my father had cancer in the glands between his lungs. On Friday, July 26th, my father went to the lab for blood work and on Saturday, July 27th he had a CT scan of his abdomen which yet again, confirmed cancer in part of the lining of his stomach as well. They also found that he had an abdominal aortic aneurysm in his stomach. Our heads were spinning! This was all happening so fast. It was like a bad dream. How could he be this ill when prior to this he had no symptoms? My father had a chest X-ray done the summer before as a check up and it was negative. His doctor even had the pathologist pull up the prior X-ray and read it again to see if they had missed anything previously but they hadn't. This was just the beginning of our education on cancer and how insidious this disease is.

Diagnosis

My father was scheduled to go back to the oncologist on Friday, August 2nd to confer on a definite diagnosis and consult as to a course of treatment. We knew it wasn't good because his family doctor had already clued us in. However, we needed to speak to the oncologist to find out the specifics. The diagnosis was specifically Adenocarcinoma of the lungs. It was already in stage three and the grade was high and considered aggressive. The oncologist advised us that this type of cancer wasn't curable but it was treatable. He wanted my father to have one more test which was a sonogram of his gall bladder. The doctor was trying to find a point of origin because evidently when you have cancer there has to be a point of origin as to where the cancer originated. So, on Tuesday, August 6th my father had a sonogram of his gall bladder and the results were negative. However, they never found the point of origin. They only guessed that it began in the lungs as the oncologist explained to us that many times a point of origin is never found. I never understood what the difference was whether or not you know where the cancer started. The point is you have it regardless of where it originated. Knowing where it did or didn't start from doesn't mean a damn thing and doesn't change anything. You still have cancer!

By this time, I was researching any information I could find about this disease on the internet and began realizing that the prognosis was not good. There was not a good rate of recovery or survival. A very small percentage of people survived. I just tried to put it in the back of my mind. I guess I tried to convince myself that this just wasn't happening.

The oncologist decided that my father would be given a course of chemotherapy to try and shrink the cancer which was scheduled to start within a couple of weeks. It would be a regimen consisting of six treatments with three week intervals. The chemo would be administered through an intravenous drip, for a few hours, right in the doctor's office. Oh yes, doctors even have a chemo room where you can sit and watch TV or movies while they slowly drip the poison into your system. That's exactly what it is, _Poison!_ The oncologist advised us that he would check my father's progress by sending him for a follow up CT scan after the third chemo treatment, which would be halfway through his treatment plan. This would be done to monitor how the chemo was affecting the cancer, hopefully shrinking it and/or putting it into remission.

Blood Pressure

Well, now we hit a bump in the road or so to speak a giant pothole. On Friday, August 9th, around 1:00 AM in the morning, my daughter had just come home from being out with her friends. She came into my bedroom and woke me up to tell me my mother had called up to her and asked her to wake us up to go downstairs because my father was not feeling well. So, my husband and I jumped out of bed and when we went downstairs my father was just sitting at the kitchen table. My mother informed us that my father had gotten up out of bed because he said he didn't feel well. She had gotten up with him and made him a cup of tea and then she said he started feeling weak and faint. I was trying to ask him what was wrong but he wasn't very coherent. He was kind of huffing and making weird noises and we really thought he was having a stroke. I told my mother to get dressed while I was trying to talk to my father and at the same time my husband was dialing 911. Then my husband and I ran upstairs to get dressed because we knew we would be going to the hospital.

When the ambulance arrived, they brought in the stretcher so fast that they gouged a hole in the wall coming in through the doorway. They took my father's vitals and even though he had kind of revived a little bit and was becoming coherent, the EMT's couldn't get a blood pressure reading. They worked on him in the house to stabilize him before they would even move him out to the ambulance. My father whispered to me that he needed to go to the bathroom but they wouldn't even let him get up out of the chair for fear he would pass out or collapse. After a short time, they put my father on the stretcher and moved him out into the ambulance. However, they continued to work on him outside the house for about ten minutes longer to make sure he was stable enough before they would even move the ambulance to proceed to the hospital. Even though our family doctor was affiliated with another hospital, the EMT's insisted on bringing him to the nearest hospital since they felt his condition was critical.

There were two ambulances that came. My mother rode in the ambulance with my father and the other EMT let me ride in his ambulance. My husband and my daughter followed in our car. My son was not home and didn't have a cell phone at that time, so we couldn't call him to let him know what was going on. We left him a note on the kitchen table letting him know what had happened and where we were. We all really thought my father was going to die that night. My mother was convinced they were going to come out of the emergency room and tell us that my father was dead. She was even trying to prepare me, telling me this might be it. Since the previous testing had also showed that my father had the aneurysm in his stomach, we thought it might have been possible that it had ruptured. But, really at this point, we didn't know what to think or what to expect.

In the meantime, my daughter had gotten so nervous with everything going on and being in the emergency room that she felt faint, so my husband bought her a soda and took her outside for some air. I finally convinced him to just take her home. When they got home, my son was also just arriving home. When he found out what happened, he wanted to come to the hospital, so my daughter stayed home and now my husband came back to the hospital with my son. I had also asked my husband to bring back sweaters for my mother and I, which he did, because it was so cold in the hospital and we were freezing.

Thankfully, they had finally stabilized my father and we were now allowed to go in and see him. They let us go into the emergency room to see my father a couple at a time. It was obvious that they were going to keep him and admit him into the hospital. So, after my husband and son had gone in to see my father, I told them to go home and said that my mother and I would stay in the emergency room with my father. I told my husband I would call him in the morning and let him know what was going on. There was only one chair by my father's bed in emergency, so my mother sat on the chair and I sat on the floor until finally a nurse came by and brought me a chair to sit on. All I remember is that it was freezing in there but we just wanted my father to feel secure in knowing we were there with him. It was not a pleasant night sitting there watching him and all the monitors he was hooked up to. Afterward, he said that all he remembered was a lot of people standing over him and working on him with all the machines around, getting all his vital signs stabilized.

This particular hospital is notorious in testing for heart problems, since they have added a new cardiac wing. Stories have been told of people going in the hospital for one illness only to be told they have heart problems when they really don't. Keeping that in mind, during the course of the night, one of the attending physicians came in to check on my father. He said and I quote, "Maybe we have to do catherization or maybe put in a pacemaker." At the same time, my mother and I both jumped at him and said, "Oh no, he doesn't have a heart problem and we will have our family physician decide on what testing he may need!" With that, the doctor just backed off and said, "Okay, okay." No matter what you read through the rest of this book, my father never had and never developed a heart problem. It's so crazy because you really have to be aware and on top of things because if your illness doesn't kill you, in my opinion, a doctor or hospital may!

In the morning, I called my husband to come back to the hospital and pick up me and my mother so we could go home for a while, eat something and take a shower before returning back to the hospital. We had given my father strict instructions that if any doctors came in and wanted to do any testing or procedures of any kind while we were gone, he was to say no, not sign for anything and tell them to call us first. We weren't taking any chances. When we got back to the hospital, my mother and I decided to call my father's medical doctor to let him know my father was in the hospital. However, the doctor was on vacation, so the service said they would beep the doctor on call and have him call me on my cell phone in the hospital. A few minutes later, my mother noticed two doctors sitting at a table in the emergency room going over charts and she noticed that one of them was the doctor we were trying to contact. She had gone to him once before when her doctor was on vacation, so she knew who he was. I walked over to him and explained who I was and the situation we were in with my father and at the same time I was speaking to him he was getting the beep from his service to call me.

Anyway, he came right over to my father to assess the situation and checked his chart. We told him what had taken place and also advised him about the emergency room doctor telling us my father may need catherization and a pacemaker. He said not to worry and that he would handle it. He then asked me why they were giving my father Pepcid. During the course of the night, the nurses kept coming in and giving him all kinds of pills, some of which were Pepcid. I told him I didn't know but it was a good question, since he was not having any stomach problems. Once again, he said not to worry, he would take care of everything.

Since there were no rooms available at that time, they temporarily put my father in what they call a holding area at the end of the hallway until such time as a bed would become available. However, after some general testing, they still could not find a reason why his blood pressure had dropped so severely and while he was in the hospital; of course, his blood pressure was remaining stable. So, they released my father that afternoon, Friday, August 9th with no significant findings.

The next day, Saturday, August 10th, I was monitoring my father's blood pressure. I have a blood pressure machine at home, since I have high blood pressure and check my own pressure from time to time. My father's pressure was starting to drop again and now he was breaking into a sweat and starting to feel weak. We made him lie back and put his feet up in the recliner chair he was sitting in and gave him orange juice. We also took his temperature which was now about one hundred degrees. We figured he must have some kind of infection going on in his system since he was starting to run a fever. However, after a few minutes, his pressure slowly started to return to normal.

My father's medical doctor was still on vacation, so I called and spoke to the doctor on call again to explain what was happening with my father and see what he could recommend to us. The doctor advised us to stop my father's blood pressure medication for now, which under normal circumstances he took for high blood pressure and also advised us to give him Gatorade for the weakness. The doctor explained that the electrolytes in the Gatorade would also bring up my father's blood pressure. I asked the doctor's opinion about a possible infection since he was starting to run a low grade fever and he told me it could be possible. The doctor told me to call and advise him if my father's temperature went up higher than one hundred degrees. So, during the next few hours, we kept checking his temperature as well as his blood pressure. When my father's temperature reached one hundred and one degrees I called the doctor again, who then prescribed an antibiotic also believing that there had to be some kind of infection going on in his system as well. A few months down the road, we were educated to the fact that when you have cancer, you can also run fevers. However, at that time, no one was sure or could advise us exactly what was causing the fevers.

Even though we followed the doctor's orders and did everything we could, during the course of the weekend, my father's blood pressure still kept dropping from time to time. So, on Monday morning, August 12th, we made the decision to call an ambulance and have him brought back to the hospital again. This time, we requested that the ambulance bring my father to the hospital where his doctor was affiliated. Something was obviously wrong and we needed to find out what kept causing his drop in blood pressure. While my father was in the hospital, they still could not determine a reason for his drop in blood pressure and once again, while in the hospital, his pressure had stabilized.

This time, we called the oncologist to also let him know what was taking place. He came in to check my father as well and while my father was in the hospital, the oncologist decided to administer my father's first chemotherapy treatment to get him started. So, on Wednesday, August 14th, my father had his first round of chemotherapy. Thank goodness he tolerated it well with no bad side effects. I couldn't believe it. I walked into his hospital room after work and there he was sitting up and eating while the intravenous was dripping the chemo into his arm. It seemed to be okay. The chemo wasn't making him sick and he was handling it well.

My father was supposed to come home from the hospital by that weekend. However, the doctor decided to do a Doppler test on the carotid arteries in his neck. They were still in the process of trying to figure out what else could be wrong or going on which would cause his blood pressure to keep dropping. The Doppler showed that he had a blood clot in one of the carotid arteries in his neck. They now called in a vascular surgeon who ordered an MRI of his head to make sure the cancer hadn't spread there and to make sure that there weren't any other problems or complications. The MRI was negative so they prescribed Heparin, which is a blood thinner, to dissolve the blood clot. This meant that now my father had to remain in the hospital for a few more days until the Heparin was regulated to the right dosage. My father was finally released from the hospital on Friday, August 22nd.

On Sunday, August 24th, my father's temperature was up again to one hundred and two degrees. This was getting frustrating now. The next day, his medical doctor was back from vacation and my mother called to fill him in on what was happening and the doctor told my mother that after his office hours he would come to the house and check my father. You don't get many doctors like that anymore who will make house calls. Anyway, when the doctor arrived at the house, he checked my father and withdrew some blood to send to the lab for testing. When you have cancer and are undergoing chemotherapy, you have to constantly have your blood cells checked and my father had to have it checked twice as much since he was now also on a blood thinner. His doctor told us to continue the antibiotics and just keep doing everything else the same. So we continued the same regimen. When he felt weak, we sat him in the recliner chair, put his feet up and gave him Gatorade. As this was happening, I would constantly check his blood pressure to assure it was going up to normal range again. My father would call me his nurse and used to look for me and say, "Check my pressure." It was kind of comical at the time.

Chemotherapy Treatments

Until my father's next chemo treatment which was scheduled on Tuesday, September 3rd, he had some good days and some not so good days. A lot of the time, my father felt weak and generally unwell. My father was supposed to get his second chemo treatment in the oncologist's office but since the oncologist had just returned from vacation, he had double the patients scheduled for chemo so he was administering the chemo treatments in the hospital. So, my father's second treatment took place at the hospital in a designated area for chemotherapy patients. I drove my mother and father to the hospital and waited until my father got settled on the chemo and then came home. My mother stayed with him and I went back later when he was done to pick them up since the chemo treatment took about four hours. The first couple of days after chemo are your strongest, mostly because of the steroids and premedication they administer. It's almost like you're on a high, but a day or so after you crash and become very weak.

I remember one time after my father had undergone a chemo treatment, he came home and the next day he was outside trimming the bushes around the house with the electric saw like a wild man. At the time we laughed because we thought there would be no more bushes left by the time he was done. But after a while, he became tired and had to go in the house and lay down. He didn't even have enough strength to clean up the cuttings around the bushes, so my next door neighbor did it for him. Then there was another time my mother let him drive home from the doctor's office after one of his chemo treatments. He was so hungry that his appetite was ravenous. He ate so fast that we told him the fork made sparks on his plate. You couldn't help but laugh, but the next day as usual he would crash. He didn't even remember driving home from the doctor's office. So, after that, we made sure he didn't drive again.

In between his chemo treatments, my father would have to have blood work done and go to the oncologist's office for checkups. Sometimes, if his blood count was low he would need an injection. They administered an injection of Procrit for building up red blood cells and Nuprigin for building up white blood cells. It's amazing how much you learn when a loved one becomes ill. Over time, it finally got to the point where my father was too weak to go to the lab to have his blood taken, so the doctor arranged for my father to have home draw, which meant that a technician would come to the house every week to draw his blood so we wouldn't have to worry about getting him to the lab if he was too weak.

CHAPTER FOUR

MY HUSBAND'S ILLNESS

On Saturday, September 21st, my husband and I finally got the chance to take a weekend away to Atlantic City as we used to go every so often. It had become our get away. We would have some lunch, walk on the boardwalk, browse the shops and then go for a relaxing dinner and sometimes a show. But this particular weekend, while we were there, my husband did not feel well. He went up to our room before dinner to take a nap while I remained down in the casino for a while to gamble. When I went back up to the room, my husband was all clammy and sweaty and I could tell he had a fever. So, I gave him some Tylenol and he went back to sleep for a while. When he woke up he was feeling a little better and we went to dinner and then to the casino again. We went home the next morning and he was still feeling kind of crappy.

During that week, my husband still wasn't feeling that well and kept running a low grade fever on and off. I finally convinced him to go to the doctor and get it checked out. The doctor said it was probably a virus which was going around and advised it would just have to run its course. However, my husband continued to break out in a sweat from time to time and was still not feeling well. I remember he had called me at work one day that same week to tell me that he felt like he was having trouble eating his lunch and that it felt like the food was coming back up on him. I could hear a little bit of panic in his voice for the minute but I told him to relax and after we spoke a few minutes he said that the feeling was subsiding. My husband had a history of acid reflex for which he took medication regularly. Generally, if he ate too much or something didn't agree with him, he would get bad acid reflux, so we weren't that concerned, since it occurred from time to time. Also, he had gone for an endoscopy less than a year earlier and everything had been fine.

In the meantime, my father was supposed to have his third chemo treatment on Tuesday, September 24th but it was cancelled and scheduled for the following week because the doctor said his red blood cells were too low and he needed to build them up a little more. My father was disappointed because all he wanted to do was get all the treatments over with and get on with his life. Finally, on Tuesday, October 1st, my father went to the oncologist's office and had his third chemo treatment administered.

On Wednesday, October 2nd, my husband had gone to bed early as usual because he got up for work every morning at 5:15 AM. But that evening, he woke up about 11:00 PM and was complaining of stomach pain which was radiating from his stomach up into one side of his chest. First we thought maybe it was gas pains, so I gave him an antacid. Then we thought that maybe the Advil he was taking all week for his fever could have aggravated his stomach, so I also gave him some yogurt figuring it might soothe his stomach pain. Now he was pacing the floor in pain so my daughter got nervous and went downstairs and alerted my mother. I also called my son on his cell phone to come home because now I was thinking that my husband's symptoms were indicative to that of a heart attack, so if I had to take him to the hospital or call an ambulance, at least my son would be home to help.

But, after a while, the pain started to pass, he felt better and finally went back to sleep. My mother and I had both told him not to go to work the next day, but of course being stubborn and very conscientious of his job he got up and went to work the next morning anyway. He felt fine all day until he came home. When he walked through the door, he told me that as soon as he had gotten off the bus and started to walk up our block, the pain started again, only this time it was on the other side of his stomach and chest. Well this time we weren't waiting. Our family doctor, who was the same doctor my mother and father used, had office hours that evening. I called his office, explained the situation and the doctor told me to bring my husband right in. Coincidentally, my mother was at the same doctor's office getting her check up so I had my daughter go downstairs and stay with her grandfather to make sure he was okay while I took my husband to the doctor since my son was still at work. The doctor did a cardiogram on my husband right in his office which turned out to be fine. No heart attack. The doctor then proceeded to examine my husband, feeling around the stomach area where he said he was in pain. The doctor stated that he wasn't sure what it was because some of the symptoms resembled that of gall stones and some of the symptoms resembled pancreatitis.

Emergency Room

The doctor suggested we take my husband to the emergency room and advised that he would call ahead and order an X-ray and a sonogram. The wait in the emergency room seemed like forever. They finally took my husband into the emergency area where you can only visit ten minutes out of every hour. By that time, my son had come home from work only to find out the situation and then came to the emergency room to stay with me. After a couple of hours, they still had not done any tests and it was getting late so the nurse suggested we go home for a while and she gave me the number of the nurses' station to call so I could find out when my husband was done with the testing. We figured he would be released after the tests were done. So, my son and I came home for a while, got something to eat and then decided just to go back to the hospital without calling the nurses' station.

As my son and I were sitting in the emergency waiting room we heard a voice over the PA system in the hospital paging my name to go into the emergency room area. When I went through the doors to emergency a doctor was waiting there for me and told me that my family doctor was on the phone and wanted to speak with me. I knew this couldn't be good. When I got on the phone, my doctor told me that he wanted to admit my husband into the hospital and that he had ordered a CT scan because the sonogram showed an abnormality of his liver. When I questioned the doctor as to what it was, he just said it was very serious. My head was again spinning. I don't know why but I came right out and asked the doctor, "Is it tumors??" The doctor just said that they weren't sure but that there was an abnormality and would know further after more testing. Looking back afterwards, I realized that my doctor must have known the situation but didn't want to tell me until he was sure. After all, he was already treating my father as well.

When I gave the phone back to the house doctor, his back was to me and for a minute I hesitated and listened to his conversation with my doctor on the phone. All I remember hearing is the emergency room doctor asking my doctor on the phone, "What did you tell his wife?" Oh my God, it had to be something bad or else why would he say that? Now I had to compose myself and go explain to my husband that the doctor wanted to admit him and had ordered a CT scan. I told the house doctor that I wasn't sure what to say to my husband because I didn't want to alarm or scare him, so the doctor said he would come with me and I asked him not to let on that it could be anything serious.

When I saw my husband, I remained calm and explained to him that the doctor ordered a CT scan and wanted to admit him because they thought they saw an abnormality on the liver but I tried to down play it so as not to panic him. By now it was about 2:00 AM in the morning. They were going to do a CT scan right away and then move him into a room. The nurse came while I was still there and gave him the liquid he needed to drink to prepare for the test. So my husband told me to go home and I told him to call me when he got settled into his room. I kissed him goodnight and left.

As I walked through the doors to come back out into the waiting room my son was standing there waiting for me. He could tell by my face that something was wrong and asked me what was going on. I just looked and him and fell back against the wall. I told my son, "Something is really wrong, I'm not sure what it is but I know that something is very wrong." I explained to my son what I knew so far and at that point I think the two of us were just a little shocked and confused.

We both came home exhausted, scared and worried not knowing quite what was going on yet. My mother and daughter were waiting for us at home and when I explained the situation to them, I told my mother not to say anything to my father so as not to upset him. He was sick enough and battling his own illness. All we could do now was wait until we got the test results. My husband called me around 3:00 AM to let me know he had taken the CT scan and was now settled into a room. I told him to try and go to sleep and that I was going to sleep and would see him in the morning.

Devastating News

My husband called me about 8:00 AM the next morning and told me that our medical doctor had come in and given him the results of the test. He said the doctor told him he had tumors on his liver and was going to schedule him for a biopsy. For the minute, I couldn't comprehend what he was saying. How could this be happening? My father is going through this, not my husband too! I told my children and then called my mother to come upstairs and when I told her, she just sat there with her mouth open. This was insane! I had my family doctor paged at the hospital because I needed to know exactly what was going on. He called me right back and told me that my husband had multiple tumors on his liver and since it was Friday, he was trying to schedule a biopsy to be done that afternoon so that we wouldn't have to wait all weekend until Monday to have it done.

I told my daughter to stay home and again, my son and I went to the hospital. It was Friday, October 4th. I called my boss to explain what was going on and that my husband was very sick and told him I wouldn't be in the office. He was very sympathetic and told me to take care of whatever I needed to do. Of course, he was also aware of the situation with my father's illness.

I had to really be strong because if I lost it now, it would not be good for anyone. So, when I got to the hospital, I asked my son to wait in the hall a minute and I walked into my husband's room and he looked at me and started crying. I just went over and hugged him and told him I loved him and that everything would be okay. But, nothing would ever be okay again.

Our family doctor met us at the hospital. They were able to schedule my husband for his biopsy that afternoon. When I went out into the hallway to speak to the doctor, I asked him what was going on. I could see in his eyes that it wasn't good. He explained that it was *Cancer* (that disgusting word again) and that it was inoperable because there were just too many tumors on the liver. The only option was chemotherapy and possibly radiation. My only words were, "My father and now my husband too?" He has been our family doctor since I was twelve years old and I know how hard it was for him to even tell me. He couldn't believe it either. Our family as we knew it was falling apart.

I don't know what I was feeling at this point except that I felt like I was floating. This was now becoming unreal. My son and I decided that we were not going to say anything negative to my husband just yet. We just told him that we would wait and see what the results of the biopsy would show. Now I also had to go home and tell my daughter that her father was now very sick as well as her grandfather. How could my children bear all this?

So, the inevitable happened. We got the results of the biopsy and it was confirmed that it was definitely cancer. My husband now knew that he was going to have a battle on his hands just like my father. He was released from the hospital the same day and now had to go through a battery of tests, just like my father did, to see if his cancer had spread anywhere else.

Our family doctor wanted my husband back in his office on Tuesday, October 8th for blood work. Just like my father, blood work would have to be done on a routine basis through the lab, but the doctor wanted to do the first one in his office. That very same day, my father was having his check up CT scan. He was now half way through his chemo treatments. We used to pass each other coming and going between all the doctors' appointments and testing. I can't remember exactly, but I think we got the results of my father's CT scan within a day or so. It was good news! The cancer was shrinking and the chemo was working. I told my husband, "See, that will be you too."

My husband was scheduled for a cat scan of his lungs on Thursday, October 10th. The results, once again were positive. He had multiple tumors in both lungs. By this time, my husband was now having trouble eating. Every time he ate, he would get the dry heaves a few minutes later. Between myself and my children, we would take turns and one of us would meet him in the bathroom with a bottle of coke syrup. That's the only thing that seemed to soothe and relieve his stomach and nauciousness.

On Tuesday, October 15th our family doctor, who is also a gastroenterologist, performed an endoscopy with a biopsy of the tissue from my husband's stomach and esophagus. I sat in the waiting area by myself (I wouldn't let either of my children come with me) not knowing what I was facing and fearing what the results would be. As the doctor came out to tell me the results, I could see once again by the look on his face that the news again wasn't good. I was about to be hit with devastating news. The doctor confirmed that my husband also had cancer in his stomach and in his esophagus which was already half way blocked with the cancer. That's why he was having trouble eating and swallowing. I asked the doctor what could be done and his response was chemotherapy. But he also informed me that if the chemo didn't work and my husband still had trouble eating, they would then have to insert a feeding tube. He also said that things did not look promising. I asked the inevitable question, "How long does he have?" At first he wouldn't give me a direct answer and just said that they do a lot with chemotherapy now. I looked at him and said, "You know me a long time, tell me the truth, what is your opinion?" His reply to me was, "Six months." Oh my God! I sat there in shock, disbelief and I think I was numb. I heard the words and knew what was happening but it just seemed so unreal. This had to be a bad dream.

I asked the doctor to please not tell my husband how bad it was, especially the part where he might need a feeding tube. I knew my husband would panic just at the thought. I told the doctor that, if my husband believed he had a chance, then he would fight. I wanted to at least give him that opportunity. He needed to have hope and a fighting chance. So, while my husband was in recovery, I sat in the waiting room and cried. No one knew what to say to me. The nurses came out and asked if I was okay and made sure I was alright. I had to compose myself before my husband was ready to leave and go home. So, once again, he came out of the test and knew the results weren't good but I just reassured him that with chemo there was hope. We still had to go to the oncologist for a consultation. After all, my father was going through it, and my husband was a lot younger so I tried to reassure him that he would have a chance as well.

When we came home, my son was at work and my daughter was in school (college) so I went downstairs and without my father hearing, I told my mother the situation and she just couldn't believe it. I told her, "six months" but we were never to say that to anyone else. We just told my father that my husband was very sick and also had to have chemo as well. He just shook his head and couldn't believe it either. When my children came home, I sat them down and told them that their father's illness was very serious but that there was hope and he was going to have chemo just like their grandfather. They both just looked at me with tears in their eyes. There was nothing anyone could say.

CHAPTER FIVE

CHEMOTHERAPY TREATMENTS

The next months would be a living hell. I am a Christian, but I truly believe that there is no hell when you die. I believe we are living it here right here on earth.

On Wednesday, October 16th, my husband had his first consultation with the oncologist. He was the same oncologist who was also treating my father. He explained that my husband's cancer was not curable but treatable. Yea right, here we go again. The doctor suggested an aggressive form of chemotherapy. My husband was to stay one week in the hospital (five days) with a constant intravenous drip of chemo, twenty-four hours a day for the full five days and then three weeks later, the same treatment repeated in the hospital again for another five days. So, on Friday, October 18th, we went to the hospital for my husband's preadmission tests and on Monday, October 21st, he was admitted into the hospital for his first week and first round of chemotherapy. My husband was so nervous the first day in the hospital that when the oncologist came in to check on him before they started the chemo, his pulse and heart were racing. The doctor reassured him that they would give him premedication in the intravenous so that he wouldn't be sick or nauseous from the chemo. You couldn't blame him; after all, the unknown is always scary especially when you are seriously ill. My husband actually handled the chemo pretty well, considering it was constantly flowing through his veins the whole week. It was a mixture of three difference chemo medications. Sort of a chemo cocktail!

During the week he was in the hospital, my husband had a multitude of visitors, including family and friends as well as his boss and some of his co-workers. We did have a lot of support. I was working three days a week at the time, so on my days off, I would go to the hospital and stay all day and on the days I worked I would go straight to the hospital right after work. At least it was convenient since the hospital was only a few blocks from my job. I ate in the hospital cafeteria many times during that week and between my husband and my father, many weeks to come.

Also, while my husband was in the hospital having his chemo, my father developed the gout in his foot which was very painful and had to walk on crutches and take medication to clear it up. Does everything always have to happen at once? All these little problems would pop up along the way and add extra worry and concern. Why couldn't it ever be easy?

On Wednesday, October 23rd, while my husband was still in the hospital having his first chemo treatment, my father was having his fourth chemo treatment in the doctor's office. My mother finally got a chance to go to the hospital to visit my husband since my father's treatment took about four hours. She left my father at the doctor's office and went to the hospital and stayed and visited with my husband for a while since I was at work.

My husband was released from the hospital the afternoon of Friday, October 25th. Upon his release, he was given a few medications to take at home. Compazine, in case he felt nauseous and steroids, as it was explained, to keep his lungs clear and working. My mother and I now had both our husbands home, both battling cancer and both having chemo treatments at the same time. What was happening here was crazy. No one could believe what we were going through.

The only good thing was that now my husband was able to eat and swallow food without problems. Thank God for that much. He would never need a feeding tube. However, chemo kills your appetite so the doctor now had to prescribe an appetite enhancer called Megace. My father was also taking it for his appetite as well. At least it worked and their appetites returned to normal for a while. Oh, but wait, a few days later, my father and my husband both broke out with sores in their mouths from the chemo so the doctor now had to prescribe a mouth rinse to heal the sores. What a trip! Neither one ever caught a break.

During the month of November, one of my uncles was also diagnosed with cancer having a tumor in his lung which was inoperable because it was too close to his heart. After the holidays, my uncle would also start his battle having both chemotherapy and radiation treatments. There would be no end to our family's anguish.

Thanksgiving Holiday

The week of November 18th (one week before Thanksgiving) my husband was admitted to the hospital for his second round of chemotherapy. This time, he was a little more at ease since he now knew what to expect. We were even getting to know the hospital staff. The nurses were all very accommodating and it got to the point where I would just go down the hall to the utility room myself to get any supplies he needed for his room, such as water, tissues, etc.

My husband was looking forward to Thanksgiving. Thanksgiving was always at our house with my father's side of the family and this year everyone volunteered to cook something to bring so that my mother and I wouldn't have the burden to cook and prepare everything ourselves since we were so busy and tired with everything else that was going on in our lives. However, Thanksgiving was a mixed blessing. We were glad to have my father and husband home but my father fared much better that day than my husband. Thanksgiving day my father felt pretty good. He was able to eat and stay up and pretty much enjoyed the day. My husband, on the other hand, was not as fortunate. He was having a rougher time in that he was very tired and didn't have a good appetite. He was starting to feel the after effects of the chemo from the week before. I remember he was so frustrated. I told him to go lie down and sleep for a while before company came so that he would be rested. He had lost some of the taste of food and really couldn't enjoy the dinner which was very frustrating and disappointing for him. Thanksgiving was one of his favorite holidays. I felt so bad for him and there was nothing I could do to make it better. I just tried to be supportive and give him whatever he wanted.

Back to Work

More than anything, my husband wanted to be able to go back to work. However, he couldn't handle traveling back and forth to Manhattan via public transportation every day because it would have been too tiring for him. So, his boss set him up on the computer at home and he was able to conduct some business via e-mail and telephone and then two days a week he drove to work. I remember the first day he physically went back to work. He wanted me to go with him so we drove in together to make sure he would be strong enough and able to make the drive back and forth. It was such a memorable day. His security staff was waiting for him to address them before they started their shift. Before he became ill, part of his job was to speak to the security staff and go over the events for the day before their shift started. It was so touching. There was not a dry eye in the place. They were so happy to have him back and I remember standing in the background to let him have his glory but he brought me up to the front and introduced me to the whole staff. They all clapped and it was an incredible moment.

The museum also gave my husband his own parking space to make it easier for him to be at work. He worked short days and managed by sheer will to continue his responsibilities at work. His boss and his staff were very kind and accommodating. There wasn't anything they wouldn't do for him. By this time, his appetite had returned and he was actually gaining weight which was a good sign. It seemed like he was holding his own. His outlook and attitude was so positive that we really thought he was on his way to remission.

Clinical Trial

On one of his doctor visits, I inquired with the oncologist about clinical trials. He advised us that there was a clinical trial offered at St. Vincent's Medical Center in Manhattan but explained that my husband would have to be chemo free for at least two months in order to qualify. So, the oncologist put us in touch with the doctor in charge of the trial at St. Vincent's. We were scheduled for an appointment on February 10, 2003 to have a consultation with the doctor and were advised that we would need to bring all of my husband's medical records. I now had to go to the hospital where my husband had all his tests and treatments and get copies of all of his medical records and test results. We would need to bring all his information for evaluation and review by the doctor at St. Vincent's Medical Center to see if my husband would even qualify for the clinical trial. So, for now, we would just have to wait.

Progress

December 3rd was my father's sixth and last chemo treatment. He was so thrilled that he was finished. However, as time went on he wasn't feeling any better or getting any stronger and kept complaining that he was still feeling weak.

Then, on Monday, December 16th, the doctor sent my husband for a follow up CT scan to see how he was progressing. When we went to the oncologist for a consultation to get the results of the scan, the report showed no change. My husband was in what they call "stable disease." No worse and no better. However, the doctor advised that clinically, since my husband was eating, able to go to work and was maintaining a good attitude, even though the scan showed no change, the evaluation was that the doctor felt my husband was doing better. Actually, during the month of December, my husband was able to do some Christmas shopping with me. We went to the shopping mall a couple of times and when he would get tired, he would sit down and rest on one of the benches while I continued shopping.

During all this time, I had still been working three days a week. On the days that I worked, my husband would go downstairs to my mother and father's apartment and my mother would make lunch for both of them. She made tons of homemade soup. It became kind of a joke. My husband would ask me "What's the soup of the day tomorrow?" There were times when my father was too weak to come upstairs and my husband would go downstairs to see him and when my husband felt too weak to go downstairs, my father would come upstairs to see him. They were a source of support for each other too. They had both lost their hair and eyebrows from the chemo, but we told them that bald was the style anyway so it didn't matter. And, it really didn't.

Christmas Holidays

By Christmas, my father was not feeling well at all. Christmas Eve we went to my aunt's house, as we did every year, and my husband was determined that he was still going to dress up as Santa for the kids as usual. However, my father wasn't able to last the night. He wanted to go home because he wasn't feeling well, so I drove him and my mother home. My son came with us in case my father felt weak. I remember on the drive home my father was sitting in the front seat next to me and he was shaking and shivering because he felt so cold. He scared me because he was shaking so much. After we got him home and settled in the house he felt a little better. My son and I then returned to my aunt's house. My husband got through the night and played his Santa role. We took pictures of him with all the kids. When I look back, I don't know how or where he got the strength to do it. Once again, it was his sheer determination. Christmas Day we all went to my other aunt's house, but we left right after dinner because it had started to snow and was getting really stormy and we wanted to get home before it became too dangerous to drive.

CHAPTER SIX

STARTING A NEW YEAR

It was now January, 2003 and we had gotten through New Years', which we spent quietly at home, as both my father and husband were just getting weaker. I don't remember exactly which doctor visit it was, but on one occasion my husband asked me to step out of the room while he spoke with the oncologist alone. Usually, I was in on every conversation, asking questions, getting all the facts and inquiring as to what I needed to do as a caretaker. Anyway, this one particular time, I respected my husband's wishes and waited for him out in the waiting room. We didn't say much on the drive home but when we arrived at home my husband asked me to go downstairs to the basement with him because our children were home and he wanted to talk to me privately without them hearing us.

So, down to the basement we went and he sat me down and proceeded to tell me his conversation with the oncologist. He told me that he had asked the oncologist what he thought his prognosis was and he said the oncologist's reply was, "I don't think you are going to make it!" Then he started to cry. I couldn't believe it! My first reaction was anger to think that he had asked that kind of question without me in the room and also that the doctor would even say such a thing. My husband said he wanted to protect and shield me but here I was involved to the core, so how could he ever think he could protect me from the facts or think that I wouldn't know what was going on. I knew from the very beginning that the prognosis was not good.

While we had been talking in the basement, my father had walked in and when he saw the look on our faces he just went back into his apartment. Later, my mother told me that my father had gone and told her that we were in the basement talking and he said to her, "Something is very wrong." All the while my husband was ill we tried not to tell my father how sick my husband really was so that he wouldn't be more upset. In the beginning, all we told my father was that my husband was very sick with cancer as well.

Now, we also had to think of how we would tell our children and prepare them for the inevitable. They had also been educated to all the facts and were involved in every phase from the very beginning. They saw and heard a lot and were old enough to understand the situation. So, my husband and I called a family meeting, sat both children down and explained to them that things were not looking too promising but we were not giving up and were going to do whatever we could. We felt that, at this point, it wouldn't be fair not to discuss with them all the facts as we understood them. They just sat there very pensive and quiet and then the tears came. I know I've said this before but it all just didn't seem real.

Also, after our conversation in the basement, I told my husband that I wanted to call the oncologist the next day and speak to him directly to see exactly what the situation was and if there was anything else we could do. So, the next day, I did call and speak to the oncologist and basically he told me the only thing we could do at this point was wait for the clinical trial.

My Father's Setback

The second week of January my father developed a cough and on Saturday, January 18th he started coughing up blood, so we decided we better get him to the hospital. Once again, we called 911 for an ambulance. My daughter stayed home with my husband, my mother rode in the ambulance with my father and my son and I followed the ambulance in my car. We also called the oncologist to let him know my father was at the hospital and he said he would meet us in the emergency room. In the meantime, while my father was in emergency, they did a chest X-ray. When I asked the oncologist why my father was coughing up blood, his response to me was, "From the cold air." I couldn't believe the doctor said that to me! Just because it was cold out didn't justify my father coughing up blood. This was nuts. I'm not a doctor but I know enough that you don't cough up blood from the cold air in the winter. If that were the case, we would all be walking around every winter coughing up blood. My father had developed bronchitis in addition to the cancer in his lungs. The doctor should have just been honest. The doctor now coldly suggested to my mother that she call hospice and make arrangements to have my father put on hospice care. He gave her the phone number to call. Obviously, this meant that he felt there was nothing else he could do for my father. However, he did tell my father that if he got a little stronger, maybe they could try another chemo treatment. He asked my father if that was the case would he want to try chemo again and my father emphatically said, "Yes!" But, for now, he was too weak and wouldn't be able to handle it. My father was released that same day.

My mother couldn't bring herself to put my father on hospice care. She didn't even want to mention the word hospice in front of him because my father was still hoping he would get better. So, on January 23rd, our family doctor recommended that we get a machine called an oxygenator. It's a machine that filters and purifies the oxygen in the air and is attached to a nose piece to put in your nose (the same as you would do if you were getting oxygen). It's supposed to help you breathe easier and more comfortably. It runs for thousands of hours and you can use it around the clock, even when you sleep. They also give you an oxygen tank as well for back up just as a precaution in case the machine should malfunction.

So now my son and I had to first go to the doctor's office to pick up the slip requesting the oxygenator. Then we went to the medical/ surgical store where they carry medical supplies. When we got there, the woman behind the counter told us that the doctor did not check off the required codes on the sheet. We now had to go back to the doctor's office. (Thank goodness his office was in the area). The doctor checked off what he thought was needed and now it was back to the surgical supply store. Well, evidently they still needed more information. It seems that Medicaid does not pay for the machine if your blood gases haven't been done to check your oxygen level. Makes no difference that my father can't breathe! This is a technicality. However, the blood gases have to be performed in the hospital and my father was now at home. So I asked them at the store to please call the doctor directly because I was not going back and forth again and the doctor had told me that if they needed anything else, they could call him. They did call the doctor and the conversation went back and forth. It was decided that we would have to pay a monthly rental charge but they would give me the machine at a discounted price. So, I called my mother and said I was just going to put it on my credit card and get the machine for my father.

The medical supply store had to deliver the machine later that day, because they also had to show us how to use it and also post a no smoking sign. A sign was required to be posted on the outside door since an oxygen tank was also provided as backup in case the oxygenator machine malfunctioned.

Excessive Calcium

In the meantime, my husband was still going for blood work every week and doctor appointments at the oncologist. He was now also getting weaker and was having a little trouble eating, in that he couldn't eat a lot because nothing tasted good and he would get full very fast. My husband's legs and feet had also been swelling up and the doctor had put him on diuretics (water pills) which helped a little but they still remained swollen. The week of January 20th, my husband's blood work showed that he had too much calcium in his system, which is not a good thing. So on Monday, January 27th, my husband had to go to the oncologist's office and get an intravenous drip of a medication called Zometa. This would take about four hours, so my son dropped him off at the doctor's office and I picked him up after I got out of work.

Hospice Care for Dad

This same day, my mother had decided to call hospice because it was now to the point where she desperately needed some help with my father. She couldn't handle it by herself any longer. My father was getting progressively weaker and becoming agitated, so hospice provided a hospital bed, commode and an oxygenator (the same machine we originally had to rent for him). When you are on hospice care, you are provided all the equipment for free. Anyway, my mother explained to my father that she was getting help for him. She told him a nurse would be coming to check on him and his medications and he would have an aide for four hours a day to help get him washed and changed and do whatever else my mother might need help with. She asked the hospice director to request that the nurse and aide not mention the word "hospice" in front of my father, but just act as aides coming in to help him. They were very kind and accommodating and respected my mother's wishes. Every morning a male aide would come to the house and help get my father washed, change him into clean clothes and change the sheets on the hospital bed. The aide was a very kind and compassionate person and my father felt very comfortable with him. It also turned out that my daughter knew him as they had attended high school together.

Second Opinion

Meantime, my husband was also getting progressively weaker, so we made the decision to get a second opinion. So, on Saturday, February 1st, I called another oncologist who was recommended by a friend who had been a patient of this doctor as well. She had also been very sick and credited this oncologist with saving her life. I had called her to get his number and I took a chance that someone might be in the office even though it was a Saturday. I was lucky and the doctor was in his office. I explained the situation and my referral and he gave us an appointment for that Monday, February 3rd. I called my boss at home and told him I needed the day off on Monday because now it was important that I get my husband to another doctor as soon as possible for another opinion as we were now getting desperate.

On Monday, my son and I got ready to take my husband to the oncologist for a second opinion and hopefully more answers. My husband could hardly get dressed and I had to help him. Now he was complaining, getting agitated and upset and was arguing with us that he couldn't go because he was too weak and wouldn't make it down the steps. My son and I pleaded with him and told him we would help him down the front steps to the car. I told him this was a chance we had to take hoping that maybe this doctor could help him. We finally convinced him and after a lot of struggling managed to get him into the car. Since I had the copies of all the scans and tests which I had obtained for my husband's clinical trial, I brought them with me to show the oncologist for his review and opinion. My husband was so weak that he could hardly walk and would get out of breath. Both his legs and feet were still very swollen with fluid which didn't help either. However, the oncologist was very kind. He put the the copy of my husband's scans up on the wall and for the first time, someone was actually truthful and up front with us. He showed us all the tumors reflected in the X-rays and explained to us that my husband had very little room in his stomach because it was so full of the cancer and that's why he could hardly eat anything. Also, the oncologist said my husband's legs were so swollen with fluid that it was like carrying around two ten pound bags of potatoes all day. He informed us that he could try a different regimen of chemo and we were to go back to his office the following Saturday to start the treatment. Okay, maybe there was still hope?

However, getting my husband home from the doctor's office was another trip and a half. The doctor gave us a wheelchair to wheel my husband from his office to our car. When we got home, my husband couldn't even walk up the front steps and because his legs were so swollen, he was like dead weight. I called my neighbor next door but he wasn't home at the time. Finally, we helped my husband to sit down on the bottom step but he was barely able to lift himself up. So, one step at a time on his rear, he lifted his body up to the next step and then my son and I helped him lift each leg up, one at a time, onto the next step until we got him to the top of the stairs. The only problem was, when he got to the top of the steps, he couldn't stand up and we were afraid we were going to hurt him if we tried to lift him up. What a scene. So my husband actually crawled on the front porch back into the house. When he got into the front hall he could hardly breathe and said he felt like he was going to have a heart attack! So I told him to sit still a few minutes right on the floor in our hallway and rest a minute while I told my son to go downstairs and bring up the spare oxygen tank my mother had for my father. With all the commotion, my mother came up to see if we needed any help. We gave my husband the oxygen and when he caught his breath he was able to make his way into the living room and onto the couch. It was so sad to watch him in this condition.

When my neighbors came home and saw that I had called them, they called me to see if everything was okay and when I explained what had happened they came over to visit with us for a while.

My husband remained in the living room for the night. He had to sleep on the couch because he was too weak to get up. I actually had to give him a cup to urinate in because he could not even get up to go to the bathroom. The next morning, I called my boss and told him I needed the rest of the week off because there was no way I could leave my husband home alone with the condition he was in. Once again, my boss was very accommodating and understanding.

That same morning, my husband was able to get up enough strength to move himself up from the living room couch and make it to the bedroom to get into bed. He remained in bed the rest of the week except to be able to get up to go back and forth to the bathroom. Even that took a lot of effort as he would hold on to the walls as he walked because he was so weak and unsteady and would actually get out of breath just from walking those few steps.

Blood Transfusion

On February 4th, the doctor called to advise that my father's blood work showed that his blood count was so low that he needed a blood transfusion. So, the next day, February 5th, my father was brought to the hospital by ambulance and admitted since he would have to stay overnight to have his blood transfusion. My mother wanted to stay with him overnight in the hospital, but I convinced her to come home and get some sleep while my father was in the hospital. She needed to rest badly. So, later that evening, I picked her up from the hospital and I told her I would drive her back again to the hospital early the next morning.

My Husband's Setback

My husband had become too weak to get into the shower, so while he sat on a chair in the bathroom, I shaved him while also trying to convince him that I could sponge bathe him in bed. He finally relented and I tried to be as gentle and as accommodating as I could. I did not want to embarrass him or make him feel uncomfortable, but he did agree that he felt better after he was washed and freshened up. That night, my husband told me he wanted to go to the hospital. He said "I think you should call the doctor tomorrow morning and get me to the hospital." He was feeling really weak and sick and I think he was scared and figured if he needed medical attention, at least he would be in the hospital. I told him I would do whatever he wanted. So, the next morning, Thursday, February 6th, I first took my mother back to the hospital early in the morning to be with my father and then I came home and called the oncologist we had consulted for the second opinion and I told him that I didn't think my husband was going to make it to Saturday for his chemo treatment because he was so weak. The doctor agreed that I should call an ambulance and get my husband to the hospital and said he would meet us there. So, I called for an ambulance once again.

When the ambulance attendants came, my husband was sitting on the bed and they were taking his vital signs while I gave them all his medical information and background. I don't know whether my husband's heart was starting to fail or if he was about to have a heart attack or if he just got so nervous that his heart was racing so fast, but I could see the ambulance attendants starting to get concerned and working fast to get him hooked up an to an intravenous drip. They also took out the paddles that are used to shock someone when their heart stops and put them on the bed to have ready just in case they had to shock him. I couldn't believe this was happening. My son and daughter were asking, "What's going on?" I just told them to stay calm and let the technicians do their work. I told my daughter to stay home, because I knew she was upset. When they felt my husband was stabilized enough, they moved him out into the ambulance. I rode in the ambulance with my husband and my son followed in his car.

The ambulance had just reached the bottom of my block when the EMT working on my husband told the driver of the ambulance to pull over a minute. The EMT was checking my husband's blood pressure and then hollered to the driver and said, "You better put the lights on and get moving!" I couldn't believe this. My son was behind us in his car following the ambulance not knowing what was happening, meantime the loop on the intravenous bag broke so I told the EMT to just let me hold it up because he couldn't hold it and keep checking my husband's blood pressure and vitals at the same time. What a ride! However, by the time we got to the hospital, they had gotten my husband stabilized again. So here we were with my husband in the emergency room and my father in a room in the oncology ward resting after his blood transfusion.

After my father's transfusion, his oncologist went in to check him and asked my father if he wanted to have another chemo treatment. My father's immediate response was, "Yes." However, weeks before, our family doctor had told my mother that having more chemo for my father might hasten his time, but my mother left the decision up to my father. After all, it was his life and she gave him the right to choose. Maybe the chemo would start to work again. I guess he felt it was worth a try. So, that same day my father received another dose of chemo while he was still in the hospital. My mother and I were passing each other in the halls of the hospital that day. What insanity! Before they released my father from the hospital, he had been sleeping and upon waking up had become a little confused. The nurses were asking him questions before they would let him go home to make sure he was coherent, but when they asked him his age, he kept insisting he was sixty-nine. He was actually seventy-five! He seemed to know everything else but his age confused him. However, they decided to release him and let him go home. After he had gotten home, he told my mother he didn't know why he couldn't remember his age.

Well at least my father was now settled back at home but my husband was not doing well at all. His legs and feet were so swollen, it was horrible. He was now admitted back into the hospital where they continued the diuretics as well as other medications. The doctor prescribed liquids for him because at this point, he really couldn't eat or swallow solid food. He had to use a urinal and bed pan because he could not even get out of bed anymore. I thought if they could get him stabilized that maybe the oncologist would try to start a chemo treatment while he was in the hospital. He was supposed to have gone to the doctor's office that Saturday to have more chemo anyway. Little did I know! Over the weekend, the nurses actually wrapped and bandaged his legs and feet to get the swelling down. They also raised the hospital bed to keep his legs elevated. The swelling went down to the point where they were able to take the bandages off and put support socks on. After all this time and waiting, the clinical trial was only a few days away but it was out of the question because my husband was now too weak to make it, so it had to be cancelled.

CHAPTER SEVEN

THE BEGINNING OF THE END

Saturday, February 8th was my mother and father's fiftieth wedding anniversary. One of my cousins had come to visit my father at home and my parents were showing him pictures from their wedding and honeymoon. Right before my father had gotten sick, my husband and I had been discussing planning a party for their fiftieth anniversary, but now that would not be happening. However, we had given them a surprise fortieth anniversary party and had taken a video and pictures so I was glad that we had at least done that.

Terminal News

Monday, February 10th, I had to go to work because I had taken off the week before. My son said he would go to the hospital and stay with my husband so that he wouldn't be alone. If I had ever known or could have predicted what that day would bring I never would have let my son go to the hospital alone. My son called me at work around lunch time and I could hear the panic in his voice. He said that my husband was not acting right. He said, "Mom, dad told me to sit him up in bed but he was already sitting up! Something is wrong!" I told my son to page our family doctor, since the doctor was usually in the hospital at that time making his rounds before his office hours in the afternoon. I also told my son to page the oncologist and asked him to find out any information that he could and to have both doctors call me at work.

My son called me back a little while later and said he had gotten in touch with both doctors. He had spoken to our family doctor who wouldn't really say much to him but told my son to have me call his office. The doctor knew I wasn't there at the hospital and therefore wouldn't say much to my son without speaking to me first. However, my son also spoke to the oncologist who was much more direct. He basically told my son that he was very sorry but there was nothing else he could do for his father and then the oncologist proceeded to go speak directly to my husband as well. My son was in a panic at this point and also told me that my husband was asking to see our daughter. I told my son to call home and tell my daughter not to go to work in case I had to bring her to the hospital to see her father and that I would get in contact with our family doctor and then I would be leaving work to go and meet him at the hospital. I really didn't know what was going on at this point.

In the meantime, my son had called my mother to alert her and fill her in on what was going on. She couldn't even go to the hospital because she couldn't leave my father home alone. I finally got in touch with my family doctor before I left work and asked him what the situation was. He told me he was very sorry but there was nothing else they could do and that the cancer was just taking over my husband's body. I had also left a message for the oncologist and he called me back as well and basically told me the same thing. He also told me that he had spoken to my son and told him that there was nothing else they could do for his father and that his father wouldn't survive longer than a couple of weeks. The oncologist advised me that they would be releasing my husband the next day from the hospital to come home to be put on hospice care. I asked the oncologist where my son was and he said he had left the room. Now I was getting nervous and I asked, "Did he leave the hospital?" and the doctor said, "No, he said he was just going for a walk." At this point my boss was just telling me to leave and go to the hospital. I was able to contact my son on his cell phone and told him to stay put and that I was on my way to the hospital.

Facing the Inevitable

I left work in a flash. It had been snowing and was now getting icy but it didn't matter. Nothing mattered. I just knew I had to get to the hospital as soon as I could. I would have to stay strong now for my son. I would also have to face my husband with the realization that he would be coming home to die and I knew he was realizing it as well. The doctor had told my husband directly that there was nothing else they could do. My mind was reeling with thoughts as I wasn't sure what I would say to my husband when I got to the hospital or how I would act when I saw him. I'm sure at the time I was in shock at this whole scenario that was unfolding.

When I arrived at the hospital my son was there in his father's room and I asked him to wait in the hallway a minute so I could have a few minutes alone with his father. I walked into my husband's room and said, "Hi." and he just looked at me and said, "So, did you speak to the doctor?" I said, "Yes, you will be coming home tomorrow." I don't remember what else we said in those next few minutes. It's still a blank and no matter how much I try, I can't remember exactly what we said. Maybe I blocked it out but I know I tried to make light of everything so as not to panic him or, maybe, myself.

After a while, my son and I went down to the cafeteria to try to eat something and collect ourselves and our thoughts. I also called my mother to let her know I had arrived at the hospital and that I would be sending my son home. He couldn't handle much more at that point. How much grief can a person withstand in a day? After all, my kids were still young adults dealing with two sick loved ones at the same time. Their grandfather was home on hospice not knowing how much time he had left and now their father was coming home to die.

I sat with my husband in the hospital until visiting hours were over. By now, my extended family knew the situation and one of my uncles came to the hospital to visit my husband and sit with me as well, but he really didn't know what to say either. We just really made small talk.

My drive home from the hospital that night is ingrained in my head and I remember it like it was yesterday. Some things will always remain crystal clear in my mind. I cried and screamed in the car all the way home all by myself. Thoughts were racing in my head. How could this be happening and why was this happening? After all my prayers, why was God letting this happen to my family! I was yelling out loud in the car all the way home saying, "Okay God, the joke is over! Please!!! This can't be true!!!" By the time I arrived home, I had composed myself. I couldn't be a basket case in front of my children. It wouldn't be fair to them if I lost it now as they also had to cope with this tragedy happening in our family. I needed to be strong for them now.

Coming Home

That same night, one of my cousins came over and helped my children and I move some furniture out of my bedroom to make space and room for the hospital bed and all of the other apparatus which would be delivered the next day. We put some of my furniture in my daughter's room for the time being.

My husband was transported home the next day by ambulance and put on hospice care. I had explained to him that I would stay at home and wait for him since I also had to wait for hospice to deliver all the medical supplies, specifically, a hospital bed, commode and oxygenator. He was getting all the same equipment my father already had.

The next morning, everything was delivered from hospice as scheduled. The delivery men didn't know what to say to me. As much as they were kind, helpful and made sure all of the equipment was in working order, you could see they were uncomfortable. After all, they had just delivered the same equipment downstairs to my father not less than a week ago. Even the ambulance drivers had gotten to know us. They just never knew until they got to the house if they were coming for my husband upstairs or my father downstairs.

CHAPTER EIGHT

WAITING FOR DEATH

On Tuesday, February 11th, my husband was brought home by ambulance and had to be carried up the front steps into the house strapped in a chair. I know it must have been so difficult for him. My heart was breaking as he never wanted anyone to see him like that. Anyway, we got him settled in the hospital bed and there he remained. He didn't have the strength to get up or walk anymore. He couldn't even eat solid food and was barely able to swallow any liquids. At this point, all he could really manage to do was sip water through a straw.

That same afternoon, the hospital sent a hospice nurse to the house to help us with all of his needs. My husband wasn't able to use a commode since he couldn't get out of bed, so the hospice nurse explained the other options to him. He could either wear disposable diapers or she could insert a catheter. I wouldn't have thought he would opt for the catheter, but to my surprise, he did. It did make things easier all the way around, except I now had to empty the urine bag every now and then. You would be surprised what you learn to do and what you're able to do when you have to care for someone you love.

I had also arranged for an aide to come every morning to help get my husband washed and change his pajamas and bed linens. It was the same aide that was helping my father. He was very kind and compassionate and my husband felt comfortable with him just as my father did. So, here we were. The kids and I all took a leave of absence from our jobs and school to be at home with my husband, since the inevitable was only a short time away. We took turns giving him sips of water or juice through a straw to try and provide some nourishment and pain medication when needed which I actually had to administer orally dispensed as liquid from a dropper. I also had to move his legs throughout the day, to help him to be more comfortable since they were again very swollen with fluid. Actually, the way the doctor explained it was that the fluids were just gradually building up in his body and his stomach was so filled with cancer that there was barely any room to take in any nourishment.

My husband's family came to see him. His mother had flown up from Florida and his brother brought her over to see him.

Death and Dying

They say that when a person knows they are going to die, family members should reassure them that whenever they are ready, it is okay for them to pass on. So, one by one, we spoke to my husband, told him how much we loved him, assured him that we would be okay and understood that he could move on whenever he was ready.

So, having the sick sense of humor that my husband always had, he was now laying there chanting, "Okay, I'm ready, take me, I'm ready", to the point where it became humorous. One time, he even called us all into the room, myself, my children and their significant others, who were also at the house at the time, and told us he was ready and that he was seeing a white light. Of course, now we were all standing there thinking that this must be it and it must be the end. However, all of a sudden, my husband looked up and said, "Oh no, it's not a white light, it's just a white hat!" My daughter's boyfriend was wearing a white baseball cap at the time. Needless to say, we all broke out in laughter. We finally had to tell my husband that while it wasn't funny, maybe he was ready to move on but obviously, wherever he was to move on to, they weren't ready for him just yet.

My son also asked if he could sleep in our room that night, I don't remember why he decided to do that but I guess he wanted to be with me and be near his father, so I just let him sleep in our room that night.

Also, that same evening, my father had become more agitated than usual. He just couldn't seem to get comfortable. The hospice representative had told my mother that my father's deterioration would be gradual. Especially since he was still eating three meals a day and was able to get out of bed to use the commode. It was explained to us that his appetite would gradually decrease, he would become weaker and he would sleep more, etc. However, that night, he was up and down most of the evening into the late hours. At one point, he must have even gotten up without my mother realizing and taken a walk for himself, since we found one of his slippers in the basement not ever knowing how it got there.

We had finally convinced my mother that she should call hospice and arrange to have a night nurse start coming in so she could at least get a few hours sleep at night. She had decided to call the next day and see about arranging for someone to come in to help her during the night. My father couldn't help it but he was keeping my mother up all hours and it was taking its toll on her now.

Death Calls for My Father

The next morning, Wednesday, February 12th, which was also my forty-ninth birthday; my mother called me on the phone and woke me up about 7:00 AM. She told me my father wasn't doing well and that I should come downstairs. I couldn't believe what was happening. My father's breathing was horrible. He was just sitting up in bed, breathing heavy with a rattling sound in his chest and my mother was on the phone with a representative from hospice. She put me on the phone with the hospice worker who explained to me that this was the beginning of the end for my father. She asked me if I understood what was happening as she told me my father was dying. I asked her how long and she said, "It could be hours or it could be days." I couldn't believe it. He was just sitting up in the bed, struggling with his breathing and for the first time ever, I prayed for God to take him so that he wouldn't suffer anymore.

I sat with father and my mother asked him, "Do you know what today is?" He looked at her for the minute and she said, "It's Lou's birthday. Did you wish her happy birthday?" My father looked at me and whispered, "Happy birthday." Those were to be the last words I would ever hear my father say. I then went upstairs to break the news to my son and daughter and told them both to go downstairs to see their grandfather since we didn't know how long he had remaining.

My father held on to my son's hand for dear life and looked at him in a way that I can't explain. I guess he knew he would be leaving us and also knew that my husband was sick as well and was worried for all of us. You could see his concern for us even as he was dying himself. I had also told my husband that my father was dying and when he heard he just cried.

In the meantime, the hospice aide had arrived and we explained that my father was not doing well. He still helped my father get washed and my son had assisted him that morning. Just about as they were finished washing him, my father took his last breath. My mother was in the other room and my daughter and I had gone back upstairs to be with my husband. My son asked the aide to help get my father dressed before they would tell my mother he had passed. We just didn't realize that the reason my father was so uncomfortable and agitated the night before was because his body and organs were starting to break down.

So here we were, my father had just died and my husband was upstairs in a hospital bed terminally ill. My son came upstairs to get me and my daughter and we went down to say goodbye to my father for the last time. I also now had to break the news to my husband and tell him that my father had just died. His reply to me was, "Tell him I'll see him in a few days."

We now had to start making calls to the family. I didn't have the heart to call my father's two sisters, so I called a cousin from each family to have them break the news to each of their mothers. Everyone was a little shocked because they were expecting my husband to die first but not my father yet. My mother gave my father's family the option to come to the house to see my father one last time before the funeral director would come to pick up his body. One of my father's sisters and some of my cousins came to the house to see my father. When I walked in downstairs, the first person I saw was one of my male cousins. He just hugged me and cried. Some of my cousins also came upstairs to see my husband as well.

When the funeral director came to the house, he was very kind and sympathetic. He guided us through the process of what we would need to do and the steps for making all the arrangements. This would be a first for me as well as my children. Also, watching them wrap my father's body, putting him in a body bag and watching him be removed from the house was another surreal experience.

The first night of my father's death, my husband was rambling saying, "I see people." I asked him who he was seeing and he said he saw my father and his grandmother. I figured it was just his imagination working since he knew my father had just died that morning. So, I questioned my husband and asked him, "What is my father wearing?" I was curious to see what his reply would be. He responded and said, "I don't know what he's wearing, but he is reading a map and my grandmother is laughing." I guess it's easy to speculate, but maybe someday, I will know what he really saw, if anything. I just hope that after my father passed he really wasn't confused and lost and trying to find his way.

That same night, which was also my birthday, my son had gone out and come home with a dozen roses for me from my husband. He told me that a few days before, his father had asked him to do that for me.

Funeral Arrangements

We decided that the wake for my father would start the following evening, February 13th and he would be buried on February 15th. So, the next day, February, 13th, my mother, my son and I went to the funeral home to make the final arrangements. I let my daughter stay home with my husband. He couldn't be left alone and she said she would be okay to stay with him. We also had to bring clothes to the funeral home for my father to be dressed in. My mother let my son pick out a suit and a tie for his grandfather. He also picked a second tie, which was kind of a loud and busy tie, to also put in the coffin because it was one of my father's favorites. When we got to the funeral home, the funeral director took us downstairs and we walked through what felt like a dungeon, viewing and deciding on an appropriate coffin. It was unanimous. The three of us chose one we all felt was appropriate and the decision was made.

We also had to pick out memorial cards, compose the copy for the obituary in the local newspaper and arrange the funeral mass. My mother and father already had a plot at the cemetery with my father's parents, who were already deceased, so at least that was one less arrangement we didn't have to worry about.

One of the reporters from our local newspaper had previously done an article on my father a few months before he had become ill. As I mentioned earlier, he was a grinder by trade and the reporter had taken pictures of my father on his truck and had done a nice write up in the paper with his picture, using almost a full page, describing his profession and trade. When she heard my father had passed, she called my mother and asked if she could take all the information, compose his obituary and put his picture in the paper as well. My mother consented and a nice picture and article was placed in the obituaries. It's very strange to see your parent's name in the obituaries. You know it's inevitable some day, but when you actually see it in print, it doesn't seem real. Everything that was happening in my life at this point seemed like a bad dream, except I knew I wasn't going to wake up from this one. I had also explained to the funeral director that I would be doing this again very soon for my husband. He was aware of the situation and was very kind and understanding.

Our next trip was to the florist to pick out our floral arrangements. My mother picked a beautiful spray of roses in the shape of a heart. My children had an arrangement made into the shape of a giant baseball with the New York Yankees logo, since my father was an avid yankee fan and I had an arrangement made up to look like a grinding wheel with a scissor and knife made out of flowers in remembrance of his trade. It was an incredible piece and the florist did an excellent job.

I had arranged for a good friend, who has some medical background and experience, to stay with my husband the two evenings while we were at the wake for my father and my husband's brother stayed with him in the afternoon. In between the times of the wake, when we were home, we would all take turns and sit and spend time with my husband. One particular afternoon, my mother was sitting on one side of his bed holding his hand and I was on the other side of the bed holding his other hand. Keeping in mind that at this point he was in and out of consciousness, he just looked up at us and said "*MOTHER AND DAUGHTER, NO MORE SOUP!*" (I decided that this would be an appropriate name for my book.) My husband realized that we were going to both be left alone and my mother would not be cooking soup for him and my father anymore. It was so sad. My mother and I just looked at each other and didn't know what to say.

Along with my son, I asked my closest male cousins and my next door neighbor, who I also grew up with, to be pallbearers for my father. So, at the funeral mass, my son, my cousins and my neighbor all carried my father's casket in and out of the Church. There were at least eight of them altogether. I'm sure my father would have been proud as I know they were all honored to do it.

Before my father ever got sick, as a joke, he used to say that when he died he wanted a phone put in his coffin just in case he wanted to call home. We used to laugh at him, but I did put his cell phone in the coffin with him. However, I didn't know until later that one of my cousins had also bought a cell phone and actually bought minutes and put it in the coffin with my father as well. I also wrote my father a letter, the contents of which are only known to me, sealed it and put it in the coffin with him. I told my children they could do the same. I felt that if anyone needed to say any last words, this was the time to do it. I hoped it would be therapeutic and maybe give us some sense of closure.

During the wake, no one had a bad word to say about my father. The only words we ever heard were what a kind and gentle man he was. He was always quiet and polite to people and always conducted himself as a gentleman.

My uncle was also still going for chemotherapy and radiation treatments and was not feeling well himself. He and my father were brother-in-laws but were also very close. I knew my uncle was upset so I told him he didn't have to come and sit at the wake all the time, but he insisted on being there.

When I arrived home after the second night of my father's wake, my husband was still sort of in and out of consciousness and at one point loudly stated, "You can't go until they tell you it's time to go. There's a higher authority!" I was a little taken aback at what he said and asked him, "Are you talking about God?" and he adamantly said, "Yes!" Then, during the night, he was yelling, "Seven forty-five, seven forty-five." I didn't know what he meant by that, but I figured he was just rambling again. So I had just dismissed it for the time being.

Also, that night, when my husband and I had some private time alone, I asked him to send me a sign after he passed. I told him he could let me know that he was around me by sending me a white rose.

I told him that this would be our connection. I said to him, "If I see a white rose, I will know it's from you and that you're around me." I wasn't sure if he really heard me or understood what I said at the time because, as I said before, he wasn't always coherent.

Death Calls for My Husband

I had previously arranged for the aide from hospice to stay with my husband the morning of my father's funeral, because he couldn't be left alone. It was a busy morning with everyone running around getting dressed and ready for the limo to pick us up to go to the funeral home. I had spent time with my husband earlier that morning. I was hardly able to get a few drops of water into his mouth by now, but I kept trying. It was pathetic and excruciating to witness. However, I whispered to him and said, "If you can wait until I come home from the funeral maybe we could spend some more time together. But if you can't, it's okay and I will understand." I knew the end was near for him.

So, I proceeded to get dressed and ready for my father's funeral and by this time the hospice aide had arrived and was attending to my husband. I was walking back into the bedroom for a minute and as I entered through the doorway, my husband turned his head to look at me, took a deep breath and that was it! He stopped breathing! Was this really his last breath? I couldn't believe it! The aide had been standing there in the room as well. We both looked at each other and I said, "Do you think that's it?" When my daughter heard me and realized what was happening, she went running downstairs to get my son and my mother. One of my cousins, who had come in from out of town for my father's funeral was also downstairs. He had come to the house early that morning from his hotel so he could go with us to my father's funeral. The aide and I were now checking my husband's pulse and blood pressure but there was none. I knew he was gone. This was really it. It really happened. I then proceeded to close his eyes and I placed his hands on his chest. Oh my God, I just sank in the chair and cried and called his name. My children, my mother and my cousin were now standing there behind me in the room as well. This was unbelievable.

I asked the hospice aide if he could please stay in the house with my husband's body while I attended my father's funeral. I just couldn't leave his body alone in the house. Of course, he kindly obliged. I had to now go to my father's funeral knowing that my husband was at home, just having died and that I would be doing this all over again in a few days.

It was really ironic because just a couple of weeks before, I had actually commented to my mother and said, "At this rate, we are going to have a double funeral." How could I have foreseen the truth to those very words?

My mother called our family priest to alert him because he was officiating at the funeral mass for my father and she didn't want him to mention my husband, not knowing that he had just died.

When we arrived at the funeral home for my father, one of my cousins was standing in the hallway and while I was telling him that my husband had died that morning, my mother had already gone into the viewing room where my father was and informed the rest of the family as well as the funeral director. No one knew what to say anymore. They all just looked at me and cried when I walked in. How could we all be going through this?

Eulogy for My Father

My son did the eulogy for his grandfather at the mass in church. He wasn't sure he could do it and asked me if I would just walk up and stand on the altar with him for support. One of my cousins had previously asked me if he could say a few words as well. So, the three of us went up to the altar together. We let my cousin say a few words first and while I stood beside my son, he bravely did the eulogy for his grandfather as follows:

"My Grandfather was one in a million.
No one could ever say a bad word about him.
Not only was he a gentleman, he was a gentle man.
He was a quiet, humble, unassuming man
But, he always got his point across.
He was known to many different people
As many different names,
Anthony, Tony, Sonny, Tony the Grinder and Uncle Junior,
But most importantly, he was Dad and Grandpa.
His whole life he was a hard working man.

He was still working up until the day he got sick.
In the beginning of his life
He worked to support his family, but toward the end
He worked simply because he enjoyed it.
Hopefully, he is in a better place
Surrounded by all the slot machines he could ever want.
They say things happen for a reason,
So, I guess heaven must have had a lot of dull knives
That needed to be sharpened.
I know he is looking down on all of us and he is smiling,
Because the one thing he always did was smile."

I don't know how we all got through that day as I think we were all in a daze. How could my father and husband both have left us at the same time? This just wasn't fair. That afternoon, after my father's funeral, I had asked family and friends to come back to the house to eat since some of my neighbors and friends had been kind enough to send us so much food. While at the house, some of my family members took turns going into the bedroom to see my husband to pay their respects for the last time. Our family priest also came back to the house and said a prayer over my husband's body. The funeral director had advised me he would give us some time at home before he would come, once again, this time for my husband.

CHAPTER NINE

A SECOND FUNERAL

Sunday, February 16th, we had a blizzard which lasted all night into the next day. We couldn't schedule the wake for my husband until Tuesday night, February 18th because no one would have been able to get to the funeral home in the snow storm. I remember shoveling the front steps with my son. He was yelling up into the sky at God saying "Keep dumping it on us!" I think we were just numb at that point. Even the neighbors outside shoveling their sidewalks didn't know what to say to us. Two of my cousins also came in their truck with a snow blower to help dig us out.

My husband and I didn't have a cemetery plot, so when the funeral director inquired, I just told him to give me whatever space was available. There was no way, between all that had just happened plus the inclement weather that I was going to go to the cemetery and pick out a final resting place. At this point I said, "What difference does it make, we will be in the ground. It doesn't matter where." I let my son pick out the clothes for his father to be dressed in and once again, we went to the funeral home to make all the necessary arrangements. This time, my daughter came with us. Bad enough we did this once, but twice in one week was unbelievable. So we had to make decisions now a second time. We viewed the coffins once again and it was unanimous. We all liked and picked the same coffin for my husband as we had chosen for my father. Now it was off to the florist again to pick out our floral arrangements. When the girls in the florist saw us again and heard what had happened they couldn't believe it. They were all very sympathetic as well. I picked a double heart of roses, my kids had a huge detective shield made with my husband's shield numbers on it and my mother had a slot machine made out of flowers, since my husband and I loved to go to Atlantic City. It may seem crazy, but this is what you do in the moment.

The first night of my husband's wake, a very good friend of mine walked in (she was the same person who had stayed with my husband while we had attended my father's wake) and when I saw what she was holding in her hands I was shocked. Remember the request I made to my husband to let me know he was around by sending me a white rose? Well, she was holding one single white rose in a vase! No one else had known about the white roses except my mother and my children. When I asked her why she brought me a white rose she said that something told her to go to the florist before they closed because she wanted to bring me a rose. What were the odds that it would be a white one? When I told her the story she was amazed. Believe what you want, but I believe it was the first sign from my husband.

I also wrote a letter to my husband, sealed it and put it in the coffin with him and told my children to do the same. I said, "Write whatever you want to say, seal it and put it with your father." So we all wrote our letters as we had done for my father. I felt it would be therapeutic, especially for my children to be able to express their feelings and write it down on paper.

A lot of the same family and friends who paid their respects at my father's wake were now coming to my husband's wake. People were just shaking their heads in disbelief and asking me how I was still standing. I don't know how we did it but I think we just went through the motions. Even my children were strong. It was amazing that we were surviving these days.

My husband had been employed as an Assistant Security Director for one of the top museums in New York City. He oversaw a huge staff consisting of security workers and also had interaction with many other departments within the museum, most of whom were very fond of him. As I stated previously, over the course of his illness, his boss and closest staff members would come to the house and to the hospital to visit with him. Many of them called on a continual basis, checking on his health and offering moral support to myself and my family. He was so well respected that the second evening of my husband's wake, the museum had actually hired two buses to transport many of his co-workers and staff who wanted to come and pay their respects. The line formed out the door. It was incredible and looked like a receiving line. We just stood there and as everyone came up to pay their respects one of my husband's staff members, whom we knew very well, introduced the workers to me and my children, one by one. Some of his staff was so overcome with grief that the museum had to retain grief counselors for them. What a testament to their love and loyalty to my husband. It made us proud to know that he was such a well respected individual.

Even though my husband was retired from the New York City police department, some of his fellow officers coordinated a police escort and pall bearers for the day of his funeral. Needless to say, there was a swarm of men and women in blue, both active and retired who were also there to pay their respects.

My Husband's Eulogy

My son also delivered the eulogy for his father as follows:

> *"My father was a special man.*
> *He was not only a wonderful husband and father,*
> *He was a good and faithful friend to many people.*
> *No matter how big or small the problem was,*
> *Everyone knew they could turn to him.*
> *On many Christmas Eve's,*
> *He was Santa Claus for the children in our family*
> *And he enjoyed it more than they did,*
> *Because he knew it put a smile on their faces.*
> *He had a sharp wit that could make anyone laugh.*
> *Even throughout his final days, he was cracking jokes*
> *To make his family feel more comfortable and smile.*
> *The courage he showed will help us cope*
> *With these hurtful days.*
> *In his final days, I was very fortunate to be able to tell him*
> *How grateful I was to have him as my dad*
> *And even though he was deathly ill, he wanted me*

To tell his whole family he loved them very much.
He will never be forgotten, not only by my mother,
My sister, my grandmother and myself,
But by all of his relatives and friends as well.
My father was not only my father,
He was also my best friend.
He had a heart of gold and a smile on his face 24/7
Just like my grandfather.
I know we lost an incredible person,
But we can take comfort in the fact
That we all gained a guardian angel.
If you look up the definition of the word hero
In the dictionary it says,
Someone to look up to or aspire to be like
Which just proved my father was and will forever be my hero.
And dad, thanks again for everything."

My Husband's Funeral

The funeral procession was an incredible sight. A police squad car led the procession and various other squad cars blocked off the traffic so that we could drive past the house one last time on the way to the cemetery. The line of cars was never ending. When it was over, once again, family, friends, some of my husband's co-workers and even his boss came back to the house. It was a beautiful, sunny day and I remember his boss and some of his co-workers sitting on my front steps reminiscing about him.

When everyone left, it was time to take a breath and now face reality. I spoke to my boss and told him I just needed some time to absorb what had happened. I told him I needed two weeks off to get myself together and try to make sense of what had happened and of course, he kindly obliged.

That night after the funeral, my son called me aside and handed me a letter. He said, "Mom, dad gave me this letter for you before he left the hospital and asked me to hold on to it and told me to give it to you after he died." The letter shall remain personal and private, however, in my eyes, it was a most heartfelt and unselfish act. My husband took the time to write me a last letter when he knew he was dying. It is something I will treasure forever as he gave me his last words.

CHAPTER TEN

THE AFTERMATH

The first couple of weeks after both funerals were strange ones. I would find myself walking from room to room not knowing what I wanted to do first. It was almost like I had no direction. A couple of times my son caught me wandering around in the house and he would stop me and say, "Mom, stop, you're just walking around from room to room." I would realize he was right and then I would try to collect my thoughts and put some order into what chores I had to do.

I spent some time going through all the Mass cards and sympathy cards and writing thank you notes. I also found the need to clean out my husband's closet with all his clothes and some of his belongings. I don't know why. It wasn't that I wanted to get rid of his things, but I just felt like I needed some order and organization in my life. Of course, it was difficult as I pulled out clothes and shoes. I let my son pick what he wanted and the rest would be given away or thrown out. I just kept a few items for remembrance. I didn't go through all his other personal items. I just basically did the clothes in the closet. The rest would take time.

My mother on the other hand, felt the need to keep a lot of my father's clothes. She gave some to family members who could use them and some she gave away. But she held on to a lot more than I did. I guess we grieved and handled our losses differently.

I returned to work on March 10th, 2003, trying to resume some kind of normal life again, if you could call it that. However, it was easier said than done. I was left with no income but my own. Obviously, my husband's income from the museum ceased and he hadn't worked there long enough for me to receive his pension. His pension from the police department also ceased as well as all of our medical benefits. What a predicament I was in. Never in my life did I think I was going to be left the way I was. Forty-nine years old and now what do I do? The only saving grace was that we had some life insurance.

My children and I now had to apply for medical benefits on our own. It wasn't easy. I had to make numerous calls and inquiries and gather a lot of information. But, I was determined to stand on my feet and take over. I had to do it, if not for myself then for my children. I wanted to show them that life goes on no matter what. My exact words to them were, "Our lives will never be the same. It will be different, but we will be okay." I didn't know if I believed that was really true, but I only had hope.

The month of April brought my husband's birthday, two months after his death. He would have been fifty-one. He was too young to die. Then Fathers' Day came and went and we just kept busy. There were no fathers' to barbeque or buy gifts for. It was just another day for us and instead we went to the cemetery to plant flowers. How sad.

In May, things started happening in and around the house. We had termites, so I had to get an exterminator. Then we had a blackout in the area and when the electric came back on, my daughter's friend came to visit and when she rang the front door bell (which has a program with many different songs and chimes) it played the tune "Hava Negila." My daughter and I looked at each other in surprise. It was never programmed to play that, however, since my husband was Jewish, I think he was playing with us, if you know what I mean. So I looked up to the heavens and said, "Oh, no you don't!" and then changed it back to the regular default tune. I knew he was around. Then for no reason, my air conditioner in the living room was not working. When I put it on, nothing would happen. It was strange. Even my mother's door bell was not working correctly. Well, they say that spirits work through electric and if that's true, my husband and father were having a party here. However, just as a footnote, the following summer I was going to replace the air conditioner, but decided to try it first and guess what, it worked and has worked ever since, so go figure.

We still had our dog "Candi." She was now fourteen years old. She grew up with my children and was very good and gentle with them. She was like a human and was treated like another member of the family. When my father used to work in his garden, she used to pace back and forth outside the fence just waiting because she knew my father would inevitably give her a tomato from the garden. Sometimes she would just play with it for a while or else bring it in the house and lie down and guard it for a while before she ate it. Also, during the course of the day, she would go downstairs and lay down outside my parents' door which they would keep open or go in and visit with them if she felt like it. After we would finish dinner, she always got a taste of whatever was left over and when she saw us cleaning up and knew our dinner was over, she would then proceed downstairs to my parents to see what food they would give her after their dinner. She had a whole routine. After the deaths, she used to stand in the kitchen and look up and stare as if she was looking at someone and then go downstairs to my mother's apartment and look around in my mother's kitchen. It was a little spooky at times because it was as if she saw something we didn't.

In the month of May, we also received an invitation to a communion party for my cousin's daughter. My son chose not to go, so just my mother, my daughter and I went. This would be the first function we would attend alone without my father and husband and needless to say, it was a little strange. My cousin sat us at her table and when I saw the centerpiece, I was stunned for the minute. There it was, in the center of the table, a glass vase holding a bouquet of white roses! When I looked around at the other tables, there were other floral centerpieces but no one else had white roses. My cousin lived in New Jersey and had no idea about the meaning of the white roses for me. So I asked her why only our table had the white roses and she explained that her sister-in-law had ordered them and decided they should be at the main table. When I explained the story of the white roses to her, she was floored. So, we figured this was another sign proving that my husband was telling us that he was there with us that day.

I also started therapy sessions with a psychotherapist in June of 2003 to help me cope with the losses. I don't know if it will help or what to expect from it, but I know that I haven't really grieved yet.

Another milestone was picking out a headstone and the engraving for my husband's gravesite. My mother just had to order engraving for my father's stone, since their plot already had a headstone erected. They had a double plot with my paternal grandparents, who had already passed on. So, on July 26th I went to the place where they sold monuments and picked out a headstone. I actually designed it, placing two hearts linked in the middle with a rose etched on the side and engraving on the top that reads "Love is Eternal."

Now, to actually go to the cemetery and see the stone erected and my husband's name engraved on it was unnerving! Even seeing my father's name etched on his stone was creepy. Here we were, visiting two graves at the same time. All we kept saying was, "How crazy is this?" At the cemetery, we were now planting and filling in with dirt where needed. This is just what I wanted to be doing, planting flowers at the cemetery! My son also placed a baseball in front of his father's grave since he, his father and his grandfather were all baseball fans.

The First Summer

The first summer without my husband and father felt so strange. My father would always be working outside in the yard. His passion was to grow roses, plant his garden and take care of the landscaping. He was a perfectionist and took pride in caring for his home. No weeds were to grow around his plants and every blade of grass was just perfect. He was proud of the house he built. Now, how could my mother and I keep us this legacy? Of course, we couldn't do everything, especially the way my father did, but we learned fast. Over the summer, we weeded, watered and planted some tomatoes to make a little garden. It may not have looked exactly the way my father would have had it but we certainly finished a close second. My father's birthday was in July, five months after his death. He would have been 76. I miss him.

My husband used to open the pool and now this year, I had to hire someone to open the pool for me. I basically knew how to maintain it but didn't know how to hook up the filter and get it all going. You don't realize all the things you take for granted. Also, that summer, we had to put my dog, Candi, to sleep. She was getting old and had been having trouble walking from time to time, but now she couldn't walk or get up at all. When she couldn't get up anymore I knew it was time.

So, on August 15th, actually six months to the day after my husband died, I called a veterinarian to come to the house. He examined her and confirmed it was her time as he explained she was filling up with fluid. He let us have some last minutes with her and told us to let him know when we were ready. So, my mother, son, daughter and I all cried as we petted her and said goodbye and while we sat with her, the vet gave her a shot which put her to rest. It seemed that deaths in our house were never ending. The vet covered her and my son helped him put her on the stretcher and carry her out to his car. I know this may sound morbid but another dead body was leaving the house.

The first time to the Mall after my husband's death was another small feat. You would be surprised at the emotions one event can trigger, no matter how insignificant it may seem. I kept remembering that the last time I had been there was with my husband to do some Christmas shopping together when he was feeling up to it. He even bought something special for my mother, since she had also been helping to take care of him on the days that I worked. He had picked out a bracelet with amethyst stones (her birth stone). He just wanted to give her something from him personally. It had been a very touching gesture.

Psychic Reading

The month of August also brought a lot of insight into our lives. A cousin of mine told me about a psychic who does group readings. She had the psychic come to her house and said she was so good she blew everyone away. So, I decided to have a reading in my home. I had ten people attend, including family members and friends. While we were waiting for the psychic to arrive, she called me on the phone to tell me she would be at the house shortly and that she was just caught in a little bit of traffic. She had been coming from New Jersey where she was from. While we were on the phone, she asked me if my father had passed and I said yes. She explained to me that all day she was feeling heaviness in her chest and the need to sit down and put her feet up. She explained that sometimes she would actually get the physical sensations of someone who had passed and she was describing my father's symptoms exactly. I hung up the phone crying and through the tears was trying to tell everyone what she had said. When the psychic arrived and started the readings, my father was the first one to come through. It was ironic because that afternoon my mother had commented to me that my father wasn't the type to be outspoken or voice an opinion and she never thought he would come through and here he was coming in loud and clear.

The psychic asked my mother if she was going on a trip. We were actually planning a trip to Georgia in October. My mother's sister lives in Georgia and her son who also lives there was planning an eighty-fifth birthday party for her. We were all invited as well as another cousin and her husband and had decided that all of us were going to go. The psychic told my mother that my father said she should go and have a good time and to look up into the sky because the weather would be very clear while she was there. She also told my mother that she and my father were very close, like best friends, which was also true. She spoke about my father being close to one of his brother-in-laws and said my father was referring to him as "smoky" which was also true, since my uncle was a smoker. She said that my father was with his mother and that he was conveying that passing on was harder than he thought it would be.

My husband came through for me as well as my children. She told me that my husband said I was not meant to be alone and if I chose to be alone it would be because it was my decision. There were a lot of things said that were right on target. The psychic made reference to my husband's favorite recliner chair as well as telling me that he said to keep the tradition of the holidays. I had been thinking of taking everyone out to dinner for Thanksgiving instead of having it at the house and my son had been arguing with me to still have it at the house as always. I just wasn't sure how it would be for everyone and was afraid it would be too uncomfortable since it would be the first holiday without both my father and husband. After the reading, I decided to keep the holiday tradition and have Thanksgiving at the house. She gave a reading for everyone who was there and was really amazing. There was a lot of specific information for everyone and there was no way she could have ever known or guessed all the information she conveyed. She was very precise about a lot of the information given.

Keeping all that in mind, over the past months, I had always wondered about the meaning of "seven forty-five" which my husband was chanting on his death bed. My husband's time of death was "seven thirty-eight" so, one theory was that since he always liked to be early everywhere we went that maybe he died a few minutes earlier than he was supposed to! I also played those numbers in the lottery and when I went to Atlantic City one time I even found the slot machine numbered "seven forty-five" and played on it, but all to no avail.

Still, I couldn't figure out the meaning until a few months after I had the psychic at my house. One of my cousins had also decided to have a psychic party at her house. Of course I went and this time was more knowledgeable and ready to ask the question should my husband come through again. He did come through again and I asked the psychic if I could ask him a question? She said "you can ask and I will see what he says." So I asked, "What was the meaning of "seven forty-five?" The psychic stood there for a moment looking up as if someone was talking to her and then gave me a specific name and asked me if I knew who it was because she said my husband was conveying that this person had helped him to cross over when he died. With that, my cousin who was sponsoring the party started to cry and said to me that her husband (whose name was referred to) had died at exactly "seven forty-five!" My cousin's husband had died in the 1980's only one year after they were married. We couldn't believe it! Here we were all this time trying to figure out the meaning and she never associated it with her husband's death. It was very spooky and again, believe what you want, but that was just too coincidental for me.

Our First Trip

In October, as planned, we took a long weekend trip to Atlanta, Georgia. There were six of us all together, including myself, my mother, my two children and my cousin and her husband. I made the plane and hotel reservations and my cousin's husband arranged to have a limo pick us up to go back and forth to the airport.

I sat on the plane between my two children and my mother sat across from us with her cousin and cousin's husband. As the plane took off, I started to cry. It just came over me. It was the first time since I had been married that I was on a plane without my husband. Once again, this was a new experience. However, the trip was great and it was good to get away and be with family and laugh and have a good time. It was something we all hadn't done in a while.

CHAPTER ELEVEN

MORE FAMILY ILLNESS AND TRAGEDY

About a week after we were back from Georgia, my daughter was getting headaches. Not being one to panic, (it is, of course, just a headache) I kind of fluffed it off as being a usual headache we all get once in a while. I get a headache daily from the ongoing day to day worries and stress, so what's the big deal, right? *Wrong!* Remember, this is me, my life, my family and lately anything that can go wrong - does. I swear I didn't make this stuff up. Over the next few days, my daughter kept complaining of constant headaches even though she was taking over the counter pain relievers. It was to the point where she would go to school, come home and go to sleep because it was draining her and she was constantly tired. One night she sat at the kitchen table holding her head with a towel wrapped around it saying she couldn't take the pain anymore. Now it was time for concern and to get it checked out. I took her to the medical doctor and after some questioning and examination, he gave her a prescription pain reliever to help the headaches saying that it was probably due to tension and stress since he knew the family history and all that had transpired during the past year.

So, the headaches should go away, right? *Wrong!* The headaches continued, now with some nausea and dizziness and my daughter was now complaining that her eyes seemed out of focus. Okay, now it's time to go to the eye doctor. She probably has eye strain and needs some glasses.

On November 6th, I took her to an optometrist who thoroughly checked her eyes and said there was a serious problem. He explained that she had some hemorrhaging behind her eyes and fluid pressing on the optic nerve which was definitely causing the headaches. The condition she had was called Pseudo Tumor Cerebri. The only good thing about it was that it was not a tumor. That's just the name they call it. Go figure. A brain surgeon probably came up with that one! Anyway, they don't always know what causes it but it can be stress related. Isn't everything? The optometrist also informed us that if it went untreated, it could cause blindness. Okay, I'm not hearing this! He now informed us that my daughter may need to go into the hospital for an intravenous medication or possibly a spinal tap to relieve the fluid. At this point, I wasn't comprehending this because it was so unbelievable that this was actually happening. Didn't we have enough? So, the doctor advised that my daughter also see a neurologist. Well my daughter and I left the doctor's office and on the way home we were just looking at each other and laughing. I guess it was probably our nerves because we couldn't believe this.

We went home and told my mother and my son. They were also upset. I was thinking, we can't go through something traumatic again. This isn't fair. My mother called her medical doctor to ask his opinion and he advised that we take her to an ophthalmologist for a second opinion. So, I scheduled an appointment with an ophthalmologist on November 10th. He confirmed the diagnosis and sent us right over to a neurologist the same day. The neurologist gave my daughter a thorough exam and also confirmed the diagnosis. He prescribed medication for her to see if the fluid would subside on its own and scheduled an appointment for an MRI of her head for November 18th just to make sure nothing else was going on.

My daughter had the MRI of her head done on November 18th and on November 20th we went back to the neurologist for a consultation to get the results. Everything in her brain and head were fine. Thank God. So, the course of action was to continue with the medicine for now and go back to the neurologist for a checkup every few months. Everything was status quo for now.

Another Family Tragedy

The next day was November 11th, also Veterans Day. It was about 8:00 PM when my mother hollered upstairs to me and asked, "How fast can you get dressed?" When I would get home from work, if I wasn't going out, I usually changed into my pajamas to be comfortable. I went to the top of the stairs and asked, "Why?" She said, her cousin's neighbor called to say that something happened to her cousin's husband, her cousin was hysterical and the neighbor wanted to know if we could go to the house. This was the same couple who came to Georgia with us a few weeks earlier. My son had just walked out the door on his way to go out and when my daughter heard what happened she hollered out the window to tell him. He told her to tell me he was going straight to my cousin's house and would meet us there. My mother and I got dressed and arrived at the house five minutes later. They only lived a few minutes away. I told my daughter to stay home, since she was just diagnosed with her eye problem and not feeling well herself, I didn't want her to get anymore upset.

When we got there, my cousin's husband was lying in the driveway, the ambulance and fire department were already there and the EMT's were working on him. I couldn't believe what I was seeing. They were pounding on his chest and shocking him and his face was all bloodied. He evidently had sustained a massive heart attack and had fallen down and landed right on his face. His wife (my cousin) was standing there crying and rambling in shock. They had just returned home from food shopping and he had told her to put on a pot of coffee because he felt like having a piece of cake and a cup of coffee. He then proceeded to go back outside to put the car back in the garage while she was putting the groceries away and making the coffee. However, he never made it back into the house. A neighbor, walking her dog, found him laying face down in the driveway. At first she thought he might have just fallen but when she got no response from him, she rang the door bell and told my cousin to call 911. It had only been a matter of minutes. He had gotten the car in the garage but when he came out, he must have had the heart attack.

We waited while they put him in the ambulance. We knew it was bad because the ambulance wasn't leaving the house yet as they were still working on getting his vital signs. You could see the ambulance rocking back and forth as they were working on him. After a while, they were finally able to transport him to the hospital and I took my cousin in my car with my mother and my son followed in his car as we trailed the ambulance to the hospital. When we arrived at the hospital, they brought us into a waiting area right inside the emergency room while a nurse explained the situation. It didn't look hopeful. They had to keep shocking him to get his heart going and he was on a respirator because he wasn't able to breathe on his own.

This can't be happening. Not again. Less than a year, we are losing someone else. A few minutes later, we saw a doctor walking towards us. I knew the look. I could see it in his face. He was coming to tell us my cousin's husband had died. My God, we were doing this again.

Over the next few days, we attended his wake and funeral. Remember the story of the white rose I wrote about previously? When my husband is around he is supposed to send me a white rose? Well, as my mother, my children and I were standing in the cemetery, the funeral director handed everyone a flower as we approached the gravesite which is supposed to be placed at the grave after the ceremony. My son, my daughter, my mother and I were each handed a white rose. My son noticed it right away and brought it to my attention. I did not see anyone else around us holding a white rose. Every other color was around us but white. Pink, yellow, red, but no one else but us were holding white roses. So, once again, I guess my husband was telling us he was there. It had to be a sign because what were the odds that only the four of us were handed white roses!

Thanksgiving and More Family Tragedy

It was now approaching Thanksgiving time and every year I had Thanksgiving Day at my house with my father's family as usual. This year would be no different. No one expected me to have it but I had decided to keep everything as normal as possible. I wanted to keep the tradition. Of course, the first holiday without my father and husband was difficult. One of my uncles wasn't there either. He was still battling cancer and was in the hospital not doing very well. During the course of the day, my aunt and cousin brought him some food to the hospital. My mother and I went to visit him the next day, but he was sleeping.

We just left him a note to let him know we had been there. It was very upsetting because after all we had seen and been through we knew it didn't look promising for him.

About a week later, Friday, December 5th, my uncle came home from the hospital to be put on hospice care. It had started to snow and they were predicting a bad storm. It started to really get bad, so I left work about 3:00 PM. What should have been a ten minute drive home turned into a two hour trip. The roads were horrendous and there were buses stopped along the side of the road because it was so icy. I made it home about 5:00 PM and a little while later my cousin called. My daughter handed me the phone and said my cousin sounded kind of funny on the phone and just asked to speak to me. Her father, my uncle, had come home from the hospital but he wasn't home very long when he had passed away. Thank God the hospice nurse had been there with them. Now tell me this isn't crazy. We lost four family members in one year. When does this end!

CHAPTER TWELVE

RECAP

So, basically the recap is this; my parents celebrated their fiftieth wedding anniversary on Saturday, February 8th, my father died four days later, on my birthday, Wednesday, February 12th and my husband died three days later on Saturday, February 15th the morning of my father's funeral. My God, how could this be? How could we all survive this? I know we don't live forever but why were they both taken together? I don't know how we got through those days and as I look back now, some things are hard to remember and some of it will always stay clear in my mind. To this day when people hear our story they can't believe it. It almost seems impossible.

The last couple of weeks of my husband's and father's lives were the most painful. How do you watch someone die who doesn't know they are dying and how do you watch someone die who knows they are dying? It was not an easy task.

I hope when it is my time I can be as brave as they were. During the last few hours of my father's life, he must have realized he was dying even though he could not speak. It showed in his eyes. We took turns sitting with him and holding his hand but he especially held on to my son's hand and kept looking at him. His face seemed to convey that he wanted us to be okay and be brave. He knew my husband was very ill but didn't know that he also had only a short time left to live. We couldn't tell him. How could he bear knowing his only child was losing her father and her husband at the same time? Sometimes I wish that I could have time back so that maybe I could have said or done something more for them. At the time, things were happening so fast that I can only look back and think that I did the best that I could under the circumstances, as did my mother and my children.

When my father and husband both became ill, my husband and I were just starting to enjoy our lives. Not that we didn't enjoy the past, but now our future was settling. Our children were grown and we were enjoying going out to eat, going to Atlantic City on the weekends and even after twenty-two years of marriage, still enjoyed each others' company. No matter what disagreements or trials and tribulations we encountered, we always ended up friends.

Letter to the Oncologist

After everything we had been through, I was especially reflective about a lot of things that happened to my father and my husband. I was also dismayed with some of the methods and ideas of the oncologist. He had the nerve to send my mother and I a condolence note and since I was a little annoyed with him I had the need to let him know my feelings. So, on March 7, 2003 I sat down and wrote him a letter. Of course he shall remain nameless, but my letter read as follows:

"Thank you for your condolence letter. I'm sorry if you did not understand our reason for a second opinion, but I have the need to convey my feelings to you at this time.

Everyone should have the opportunity to have a second and even a third opinion when faced with such a serious illness, not having anything to do with a doctor's ability but for your own sanity and peace of mind. I regret not having done that for my husband in the very beginning. He did not want to get a second opinion because he had faith in you. I knew how serious his illness was from the very beginning as did he, but you always have hope that a miracle will happen and you will survive and go on with life.

While my husband was in "stable disease" you did nothing. He had his last chemo the week before Thanksgiving and after that you did nothing while we were waiting for the appointment to seek a clinical trial which wasn't scheduled until February. Why didn't we try something else in the meantime? That was two months of no treatment! I'm aware that the outcome would probably have been the same, but you should have afforded us the decision to either stay "stable" or try something else. I know he wanted to try, but he trusted your judgment. Also, I was the one who requested a clinical trial. Why did I have to ask you? Why didn't you provide us that information?

You came highly recommended but, in my opinion, I found some of your methods questionable. I felt that the way you spoke to me at certain times regarding my husband as well as my father, were sometimes rude and condescending. You made me feel like you were bothered if I asked too many questions.

When my father was in the emergency room because he was coughing up blood and was so weak, you told us, "You don't bring someone to the emergency room because they are weak." HE WAS COUGHING UP BLOOD! We didn't bring him in just because he was weak and when I asked you what could be causing him to cough up blood your reply was, "From the cold air." I may not have an MD after my name but don't insult me with such nonsense. My father had bronchitis as well as lung cancer! After you told my mother to put my father on hospice and I asked to talk to you a minute out in the hall, because I didn't want my father to hear, you rolled your eyes at me and said , "WHAT!" as though I was bothering you. My son was standing right there so I did not imagine it. I may not have your medical knowledge but just because you have an MD after your name does not make you any better than anyone else in this world and doesn't justify that kind of treatment.

Do you realize what my family has gone through? We fought so hard to do everything and anything we could to help both my father and my husband. My father died on my birthday and my husband died three days later, the morning of my father's funeral. My family has been through HELL and our lives have been changed forever and will never be the same.

My request to you is this, in the future when you deal with a seriously ill patient, also communicate with the family. They are the ones who are worrying, not sleeping, crying and doing everything they can for their loved ones. Answer their questions honestly, listen to their ideas compassionately, and above all, give them the opportunity to make choices, whether good or bad. Family members are just as important as the patient and should never be pushed aside or discounted."

I'm sure the letter was either destroyed by the doctor or placed in a file somewhere, however, I felt better in that I got it off my chest and was able to express my feelings.

CHAPTER THIRTEEN

THE PAIN OF LOSS

Sometimes it hurts so bad that I don't know how to take the pain away. I tried to be so strong at the time but I still don't know how I got through it. You can never appreciate life as it is when people are here. It is only after loved ones are gone that you wish you would have said kinder and more loving things. Too often, life is taken for granted.

My father and husband are buried in the same cemetery where we visit regularly. It's so unreal to go visit both grave sites. As I said previously, my son had left a baseball at his father's grave since they were such avid Yankee fans. My father and my husband were also big Frank Sinatra fans. I hope they got the chance to meet Frank and all the Yankees that have passed on as well. I'm sure that would have made their trip to the great beyond worthwhile.

What happened in our lives wasn't fair. I had to abandon all hopes and plans for the future as I knew them. My husband won't be here to see our children get married or walk my daughter down the aisle. That is something he would have relished. He was a proud father and loved our children to no end. I remember one day my daughter asked me, "When I get married, who will walk me down the aisle?" I turned to her kiddingly and said, "Not me!" She looked at me in a panic and said, "If you don't walk me down the aisle then who will?" I reassured her that, when the time came, if she wanted me to, of course I would. But I also reminded her that she also has a brother who would be glad to do the same. That seemed to calm her down. My husband also used to talk about having grandchildren some day and how great it would be and I used to tease him and say, "Don't rush the time away." I never dreamed he wouldn't be here.

Flashbacks and Survival

We got through the rest of the holidays, both Christmas and New Years. It's now January 5, 2004, the holidays are over and it's a new year. I am not feeling quite with it these days. I can't sleep at night and I'm having flashbacks of my father and husband. I keep remembering certain times of their illnesses and the way they looked. I repress the feelings sometimes, but other times I can see their faces and their looks of despair, pain and fright. As much as I am feeling the loss and the pain in my heart, I can't imagine how awful it must have been for them.

It's beginning to feel a little overwhelming. I feel like I have to hold it together for everyone else. My mother is having a hard time with depression and anger, my son has his moments of frustration and anger and my daughter just holds everything in. I have to be the balancing force. But who is the balancing force for me? I have this new life but what is my purpose? I don't know where I fit in or where I belong. It's like we're all just going through the motions of everyday living and surviving. I don't know what my life is supposed to be now and even though I still have my mother and my children, at times I feel very alone and solitary. I guess it's a little scary to think of what my future will be, especially since, as I grow older, I will probably be alone. Not a comforting thought.

I can't even pray anymore. If I try, I feel like God is calling me a hypocrite. If our lives are truly destined to go in a certain path and our destiny is already planned, then why bother to pray? If we pray for health and we are destined to die at a certain time anyway, then what's the sense in praying?

I have become very philosophical. Are we just supposed to pray for help in understanding what our lives are? That's not good enough for me. I need answers to all this as I am sure a lot of people do in their lives as well. Maybe someday hopefully, we will know the answers and then again, maybe we will never know. In the meantime, it is survival of the fittest. But, how do you continue to survive under these conditions and what is it all about? I can't just accept things are what they are.

If it's true that we are reincarnated, then I choose not to come back! I'm letting everyone know now that I don't want to go through this physical life again. If there is no rhyme, reason or purpose then I don't need it. By this time, you must realize that I am having one of those cynical days where everything just bothers me. I want so much to make things right for my family, but I don't know if I am going about it the right way or what I'm supposed to do. I've become the head of the household and I don't like it much! I have no one to lean on except for my mom, but I really think I need to be there for her more at this point. After all, she is getting older and I'm sure she is frightened at times as well. My feeling of security has been taken away, yet I still have to make everyone else feel secure.

Well, what a dilemma we are all in. This is a fine mess we were left with here. Not knowing what to do at times or which way to turn. So, if there is a God, what the hell do I do now? Somebody up there better guide me!

Then, there are times I feel like I am handling it too well and that there is something wrong with me. This still seems like it's not real, like it never happened. They were here and gone in a flash. It feels almost as if I was never married. How could all that be gone in a heartbeat?

As I am learning every day to put one foot in front of the other and go on with my life, I experience a flood and rage of emotions that I could never have imagined. Sometimes I feel like I have always been single, even though I have children to prove I wasn't. It almost feels like my husband was never here. But how can that be? All around me are traces of him. There are so many things to remember him by. It's a strange sensation. Other times, my heart aches so bad that I just cry until I can't cry anymore. It's now February, 2004 and this week will mark the one year anniversary of their deaths. It's still hard to believe. This month, we will be celebrating two birthdays. I will be turning fifty and my mom will be seventy-five.

When my father first got sick, I remember commenting to one of my cousins that I wasn't ready to lose my father yet. Then after my husband got sick and things became so much more stressful and crazy, I said to the same cousin, "I'm afraid that I am going to lose my father, my husband and after all this stress, how much more can my mother take? If I lose her too I will virtually be alone, just me and my children." It was a scary thought, to have everyone around you and then the possibility that all of a sudden they may all be gone at the same time. Thank God my mom is still here and I pray every day that she remains here for a very long time.

Special Birthdays

My children planned a surprise party for me for my fiftieth birthday at my cousin's house. I thought I was going there for dinner and when I walked in, family and friends were waiting there to surprise me. My children made me feel special in that they took the time and effort to plan a special day for me.

I, on the other hand was also planning a surprise party for my mom, since she was turning seventy-five. I booked a hall and a DJ and invited all our family and friends. My mother's sister and her son and his family also came from Georgia. It was a nice evening and my son, my daughter and I each said a few words to give tribute to my mother and their grandmother.

CHAPTER FOURTEEN

<u>REFLECTION</u>

The euphemism "stop and smell the roses" is so true. Beauty surrounds us every day and we blatantly ignore it and don't give it a second thought. Reflecting back, this was brought to my attention one day, when my husband and I got into the car to go to one of his many doctor appointments. It was a crisp, fall day and I was driving because he was too weak now. When we got in the car, he started to cry. When I asked him what was wrong, he said to me, "It's such a beautiful day, look at all the colors of everything, the green grass, the color of the flowers and the blue sky." For the first time ever, we just sat there for a moment in the car taking in the beauty of the day. How unfortunate that in our everyday lives we get so caught up that we never see beyond our immediate minutes of life. We need to see the true beauty that lies around us and take a moment once in a while to just savor and enjoy our surroundings.

I read somewhere that in order to grow, you have to let go. So I have decided that it's the beginning of a new decade for me, the beginning of a new year and the beginning of a new life. This is a decision I chose to make.

I used to feel guilty that I had lived and my husband had died. In the beginning, I even felt that my husband was mad at me somehow because I was still here and living. I guess it sounds crazy, but then sanity is not very far from being crazy. It was almost like I was being disloyal to go on with my life. Guilty if I laughed and guilty if I went somewhere and had a good time. But what am I supposed to do? I guess what it comes down to is that you have to come to terms with the reality and you have to make the decision to go on. However, it's a little scary starting your life over again.

Because of the absence of one person, life is totally changed forever, never to be the same. But, we have two missing people in our lives at the same time and twice as much to deal with. As much as I am alone and a little apprehensive about the future, I have also gained a sense of independence, strength and have become more self sufficient.

Dating Again at Fifty

In March of 2004, our house alarm was not working, both upstairs and downstairs. It hadn't been working for a while but I had enough to deal with at the time and could only do so much. Over the years, the guy that put in our alarm system would come from time to time when we needed service to the alarm. We knew him for about twenty years. He was a really nice person and we used to talk about our families and just life in general. Anyway, we hadn't seen him in years and I told my mother to call him as we needed to have our alarms in working order.

Needless to say, he didn't know what had happened in our house and was shocked when my mother told him about the deaths. He came to see her right away. I was at work. They called me at work and I spoke to him on the phone and he gave me his condolences. He said he would come back that Saturday to fix the alarm system. On Saturday, when he came back, we talked and he hugged me and asked me if I was okay. I said yes and then he asked if I would like to go to dinner sometime and catch up on our lives. He was divorced and seeing as how I knew him for so long and felt comfortable, I said sure.

We spoke on the phone a few times after that and on Saturday, May 8, 2004, we went to dinner. He brought both my mother and I a dozen roses each since the next day was mother's day. Well, if you want to know how dinner went, you will have to read my next book. To be continued (…).

ABOUT THE AUTHOR

The author resides in Staten Island, in the same house where she was raised. She lives with her new husband, her daughter and a Golden Retriever puppy named Bella Mia with plans to train her as a Therapy Dog. Besides her writing skills, she has worked for a local attorney for the past ten years.

She lives and enjoys life each day the best she can and never takes anything for granted, especially the gift of life.

GLOSSARY

Abdominal Aortic Aneurysm – a weakening of the aortic wall which causes a ballooning of the vessel.

Adenocarcinoma – a cancer which develops in the cells lining glandular types of internal organs.

Carotid Doppler – an ultrasound to measure the flow of blood through the carotid arteries that supply blood to the brain.

Colonoscopy – a medical procedure to view the lining of the colon.

Compazine – used to control severe nausea and vomiting.

Endoscopy – minimal invasive medical procedure by insertion of a tube down the throat to the esophagus for visual images and biopsies.

Gastroenterologist – a physician who specializes in disorders of the gastrointestinal tract, esophagus, stomach, small and large intestines, pancreas, liver and billary system.

Gastroscopy – procedure using a thin instrument passed down through the mouth for an examination of the stomach and duodenum.

Gout – a buildup of too much uric acid in the blood which causes inflammation of the joints.

Heparin – an anticoagulant to thin the blood to prevent blood clots.

Laryngoscope – a medical instrument that is used to obtain a view of the vocal folds and the glottis which is the space between the cords.

Megace – an appetite stimulant.

Nuprigen – a hormone which stimulates and builds up the production of certain types of white blood cells important for fighting infections.

Pepcid - treatment for excess acid in stomach and intestines which can cause ulcers, acid reflux and heartburn.

Procrit – a man made protein which helps your body produce and stimulate red blood cell production.

Pseudo Tumor Cerebri – term meaning "false tumor" due to high pressure within the skull caused by the buildup or poor absorption of cerebrospinal fluid surrounding the brain and spinal cord.

Zometa – a bisphosphonate used for treating high blood calcium levels.

www.ingramcontent.com/pod-product-compliance
Lightning Source LLC
Chambersburg PA
CBHW031246280526
45784CB00004B/1740